Doing Psychiatry WRONG

Also by René J. Muller

The Marginal Self

Anatomy of a Splitting Borderline

Beyond Marginality

Psych ER

Doing Psychiatry WRONG

A Critical and Prescriptive Look at a Faltering Profession

René J. Muller

Routledge
Taylor & Francis Group
New York London

First published by
The Analytic Press
This edition published 2013 by Routledge

Taylor & Francis Group
711 Third Avenue, New York,
NY 10017

Taylor & Francis Group
2 Park Square, Milton Park, Abingdon,
Oxon OX14 4RN

First issued in hardback 2017

Routledge is an imprint of the Taylor & Francis Group, an informa business

ISBN 13: 978-1-138-42499-9 (hbk)
ISBN 13: 978-0-88163-469-3 (pbk)

Library of Congress Cataloging-in-Publication Data

Muller, René J.
Doing psychiatry wrong : a critical and prescriptive look at a faltering profession / René J. Muller.
p. ; cm.
"Lawrence Erlbaum Associates"
Includes bibliographical references.
ISBN 978-0-88163-469-3 (pb : alk. paper)
1. Psychiatric emergencies. 2. Psychiatric errors. 3. Biological psychiatry. I. Title.

[DNLM: 1. Emergency Services, Psychiatric. 2. Case Reports. 3. Diagnostic Errors. 4. Mental Disorders--diagnosis. WM 401 M958d 2008]
RC480.6.M86 2008 616.890025--dc22 2007016070

Visit the Taylor & Francis Web site at
http://www.taylorandfrancis.com

and The Analytic Press Web site at
http://www.analyticpress.com

The task of the writer is, before all, to make you see. That, and no more, and it is everything. If I succeed you will find there encouragement, consolation, fear, charm—all you demand—and, perhaps, also that glimpse of truth for which you have forgotten to ask.

Joseph Conrad

Every reader, as he reads, is actually the reader of himself. The writer's work is only a kind of optical instrument he provides the reader so he can discern what he might never have seen in himself without this book. The reader's recognition in himself of what the book says is the proof of the book's truth.

Marcel Proust

Contents

Preface

About 2,500 years ago, the Greek physician Hipprocrates wrote, "As to diseases make a habit of two things—to help, or at least, to do no harm." My purpose here is to show that psychiatry is failing Hippocrates's injunction—first by not helping the majority of its patients, and then by harming many of them.

For ten years, between 1994 and 2004, I evaluated psychiatric patients in the emergency room at three urban hospitals in Baltimore. The last step in the evaluation was to provide a referral for outpatient follow-up. Realizing the likelihood that patients would be helped by a mental health professional was small and the chance they might be harmed was significant, I often silently hoped that these troubled individuals would find another way to fix what had gone wrong in their lives. I show here how many of these patients were damaged by being wrongly diagnosed and improperly medicated, and then fold their stories into the larger story of how and why psychiatry took such a wrong turn, all but assuring that these errors would be made.

Some will argue that the evidence on which these conclusions were based is anecdotal and does not meet the burden of statistical proof that is now the gold standard in psychiatric research. My response to this criticism is that the statistical tack taken in research on the mental disorders designated in the *Diagnostic and Statistical Manual of Mental Disorders (DSM-IV)* often fails to access (or subsequently assess) the pathological phenomena targeted for study, in spite of complex mathematical operations that yield numbers implying an objective result.

The stories told here about harmed patients constitute just the tip of the iceberg of what amounted to a 10-year observational study based on more than 3,000 ER evaluations. The failures of clinical acumen visited on these patients seem to flow inevitably from the flawed precepts and directives of the current psychiatric paradigm itself. A growing body of data is revealing that many patients are not well served by this paradigm.

Proponents of biological psychiatry often seem gripped by an irrational exuberance. They use rhetoric that looks to an endless horizon of new discoveries about the brain that promise new treatments for mental illness. The fact is that we already know enough about the brain and the mind to do psychiatry right—and to stop dinging patients with wrong diagnoses and unnecessary medication. One can believe this and still be open to a future of new discoveries that would benefit those who are mentally ill.

The text ahead pits criticism of psychiatry's reduction of human experience to biological function against the accumulated wisdom, now largely spurned, of a profession that has struggled for 150 years to understand and help those with mental illness. I have tried to balance a critical perspective with a vision for what psychiatry could accomplish were it to embrace a broader concept of who and what a person is, in health and in illness.

Psychiatry should and must be judged on what we do for our patients. Anticipating that some readers will feel that what I have written is too broad a criticism of the profession, I can only say that I recognize the valiant efforts made by many psychiatrists who, against all odds, are bucking the current trend, maintaining their integrity, and serving their patients.

I have chased four previous books to completion, but the text that eventually became this book *chased me.* Mornings, I awakened gifted with key words, phrases, chapter titles, and then the title of the book itself, as if some "Deep Throat" had come during the night. Writing was mostly a channeling of past clinical experience: listening to thousands of patients tell their stories had gradually coalesced into a larger story that itself demanded telling.

Acknowledgment

Barbara Young, who has been a psychiatrist and a psychoanalyst for more than 50 years, and a friend for more than 25 years, read each part of this text as it came out of the computer, commenting on content, style, and everything else that needs scrutiny when a project like this one is undertaken. I thank Dr. Young for her wisdom, kindness, and generosity during this time, and beyond.

CHAPTER 1

Seeing Through the Illusion of Biological Psychiatry

Between 1994 and 2004, I evaluated more than 3,000 psychiatric patients in the emergency room at three hospitals in Baltimore. Some of the patients I saw had unusually challenging problems, and their stories set me to writing a series of articles for *Psychiatric Times*, which I later collected and published as a book, *Psych ER: Psychiatric Patients Come to the Emergency Room.*[1]

Halfway through my decade in the ER, I began to see that many of my patients were telling stories about their present and past lives that did not square with the diagnoses they had been given.[2] Eventually, I realized that most of those judged to have bipolar disorder and schizophrenia—to cite just the most egregious mistakes—never did meet the criteria set by the *Diagnostic and Statistical Manual of Mental Disorders (DSM-IV).*

Listening to my patients' stories, it became clear to me what had happened: symptoms they reported were matched by a clinician to the *DSM* criteria for bipolar disorder and schizophrenia without the *meaning* of the symptoms ever being ascertained—all but assuring a wrong diagnosis. While working in a community mental health center and for a private practice group, I observed a similar mismatch between patients' stories and their diagnoses. Gradually, I had to acknowledge that, in psychiatry, misdiagnosing patients had become the de facto standard of care.

Convinced that they had a "brain disease," many of my misdiagnosed patients took prescribed psychotropic medication that was not needed, sometimes to their detriment. Most of these patients had personality disorders, used illicit drugs, or consistently made the kinds of choices that inevitably lead to erratic emotional states that produce psychiatric symptoms, especially "mood swings." I was left to wonder how physicians could have violated their responsibility to see and hear their patients correctly, and ignored Hippocrates's injunction, "First, do no harm."

Most psychiatrists are trained now to believe that human thinking, feeling, and behavior, whether normal or abnormal, have their primary origin in the workings of the brain's neural substrate. Patients who have symptoms that meet the criteria for a mental disorder will most likely be told they have some kind of "chemical imbalance" and need one or more drugs to correct the imbalance. The implication here is that they have disordered and pathological lives because they have a malfunctioning brain.

There is good empirical evidence that correctly diagnosed bipolar I disorder and schizophrenia involve a glitch in brain structure and function, though no specific cause for either illness has been established. As much as any other factor, the current crisis in psychiatric diagnosis derives from a leap that was made from the near certainty that some mental illnesses are brain disorders to the unjustified conclusion that *all* mental illness is biologically driven. If a symptom is merely the behavioral manifestation of a biological malfunction, the idea that symptoms need to be understood in the context of the patient's life—that is, that abnormal emotion and behavior point back to something the patient is doing wrong and needs to modify—becomes tenuous indeed. If biology is the primary determinant of human experience, then psychoanalytic, psychodynamic, developmental, cognitive, and existential approaches to understanding behavior are of secondary importance. Many psychiatric residency programs no longer teach these theories of the self, or include them only marginally. Responding to this gap in their training, residents in some programs have lobbied vociferously for the return to the curriculum of the dynamic and humanistic approaches to understanding psychopathology.

If behavior has no specific meaning, it can have any meaning. For a variety of reasons, psychiatrists appear to be invested now in assigning the "worst" diagnoses to patients whose behavior is erratic, bizarre, and threatening, and who are difficult to treat with psychotherapy. For some time, the figure cited for the prevalence of both bipolar disorder and schizophrenia was about 1%. After the atypical antipsychotics and the newer anticonvulsant mood stabilizers came on the market and were declared to be user-friendly, the diagnostic net was cast farther out, and those numbers rose dramatically. Surely, a self-serving bias came into play here: by calling a patient bipolar or schizophrenic, the clinician opened the way for the patient to *become an illness* that needed to be "cured" with medication, and justified downplaying or ignoring altogether the complex dynamic needs of those who would require long-term, demanding psychotherapy. Misdiagnosing a patient could make life easier for the diagnostician, but at the cost of burying the truth about the patient's life, sometimes forever.

Most wrong psychiatric diagnoses tend to stick with patients. Clinicians are reluctant to risk what they see as the possible adverse clinical or legal consequences of changing their original call, or a call made by another clinician. A particularly cruel consequence of misdiagnosing someone with schizophrenia is that the medication prescribed to quell misread "psychotic" symptoms can itself cause a *tardive psychosis*, so named because it takes time to develop.[3] This is thought to be caused by an overproduction of postsynaptic dopamine receptors in compensation for the drug's blockade of the overactive presynaptic receptors, the explanation posited for the original psychosis. Those who go off antipsychotic medication suddenly are prone to a "discontinuation syndrome," where psychotic symptoms can occur, even if the patient did not have them initially.

If a patient is misdiagnosed with and treated for cancer, a lawsuit is almost sure to follow. Yet most psychiatric misdiagnosis goes unchallenged by the victims and the courts—an irony, considering that psychiatry is increasingly thought of as a medical discipline. This happens because there is no standard a clinician is held to in justifying the diagnosis of a mental disorder. Physicians diagnosing cancer must have radiological and pathological evidence of a malignant process. Unless a patient's change in mental status is due to a physiological cause that can be substantiated by laboratory tests—as would be the case with an electrolyte, endocrine, or metabolic derangement, or with drug toxicity—the psychiatrist making a diagnosis must depend on observations of and reports by the patient, and on information volunteered by others. After many years of clinical work, it is clear to me that patients' reports of abnormal thoughts, feelings, and behavior can be "stretched" to make the diagnosis of any number of mental disorders, simply by matching their symptoms to one or another checklist in the *DSM*.

Reports of symptoms by patients are often vague and are usually taken by clinicians at face value. Few psychiatrists now have any interest in identifying the possible ways that abnormal thinking, feeling, and behavior could be due to the inauthentic and self-destructive choices a patient is making, or in looking into how unacknowledged (and sometimes unconscious) choices made long ago continue to influence a life. This is what it would be to uncover what the patient's symptoms *mean*. Instead, "meaningless" symptoms are targeted with mood stabilizers, antipsychotics, and atypical antipsychotics. I once heard a representative from a leading drug company try to convince his audience that his product was the drug to use when, as he put it, "there is psychosis in the diagnosis." Not long after that I heard a psychiatrist at a grand rounds conference say, with obvious pride, that he had a "low threshold for diagnosing psychosis." With psychiatrists and drug companies thinking in this way, the odds that patients will have their stories heard correctly are diminished.

Intuitively, one would expect that the reports of toxic cardiac and metabolic effects sometimes seen in patients taking mood stabilizing and antipsychotic drugs would have encouraged psychiatrists to be more careful about diagnosing mood disorders and psychotic disorders, but this has not been the case.[4] Instead, as more prescriptions are written every day, drug companies and clinicians who write journal articles about these drugs recommend that patients be informed of the potential risks, have periodic electrocardiograms, and be monitored for weight gain, as well as for elevation of blood glucose and triglycerides.

Usually, patients implicitly accept their psychiatric diagnosis. They are often relieved and reassured to hear that the emotional pain they are suffering is not due to any fault of their own. We live in a culture where people believe they are owed a drug for every problem, and if one is not available it soon will be. In an age of growing secularism, disguised as it is with the many faces of a false spiritualism, a pill on the tongue replaces the communion wafer as a conduit to transcendence, courtesy of neuroscience and psychopharmacology.

Where psychoanalysis once maintained that the unconscious mind ruled behavior and that only the psychoanalyst had the key to unlock its paralyzing secrets through dream analysis and free association, biological psychiatry now insists that a "chemical imbalance" in the brain causes mental illness and that only a medical doctor can write a prescription to fix the problem. Freud felt that psychoanalysis could at best transform neurotic misery into everyday unhappiness. Peter Kramer did Freud one better when he claimed in *Listening to Prozac* that some of his patients on Prozac felt "better than well."[5] If, by taking a pill, patients can get around having to find out why they feel depressed, many will choose to do just that. Most psychiatrists see this pharmacological solution as an acceptable way of handling the problem.

Our inclination toward self-deception—the lie we tell ourselves, which is usually called "being in denial"—is rooted in our need to continuously respond to a world that often does not offer us what we want and need.[6] Self-deception allows us to believe what we otherwise could not believe, so we can get what we otherwise would not have, or at least have so readily. What the French existential philosopher Gabriel Marcel said about betrayal being "pressed upon us by the very shape of our world" is true as well for self-deception.[7] We deceive ourselves about things large and small because everyone and every situation we encounter requests—and at times requires—us to do so. As a result, most people are self-deceived most of the time. We go along to get along.

Patients tend to accept the promise of biological psychiatry because it gets them off the hook as creators of their own problems, while offering a solution that does not require them to change their lives. Managed care companies and health maintenance organizations (HMOs) embrace this paradigm because treating symptoms with a pill is cheaper than paying for extended psychotherapy or psychiatric hospitalization. The drug companies are happy because they are getting rich by selling more drugs to more people all the time. And psychiatrists are becoming accustomed to the idea of prescribing pills to treat symptoms (without having to worry about what these symptoms mean) because this is the only way they can earn a living now. Their compensation from third-party payers for a 50-minute therapy hour is paltry, but turning out three medication checks an hour pays pretty well. Psychiatrists who work on inpatient units in psychiatric hospitals are also forced to prescribe medication if they expect to be reimbursed by these same third-party payers.

The notion that we believe what we want to believe has been around for a long time. Fooling ourselves can reach the level of *illusion*—a condition of being deceived by a false perception—if that perception figures prominently in what we believe and in how we live. As it is most strictly conceived and practiced, biological psychiatry has slowly but surely become not only an illusion but a *collective illusion*, being subscribed to by so many—patients, doctors, drug makers, insurers—whose needs it meets, if inauthentically. The pie-in-the-sky promises perpetrated through this illusion stretch to the horizon: just spend enough money and do enough research and every mental illness will be understood. There is something for everybody here, which is why the illusion persists.

"Every age has its peculiar folly; some scheme, project or phantasy into which it lunges, spurred on by the love of gain, the necessity of excitement, or the mere force of imitation." So noted Charles Mackay in *Extraordinary Popular Delusions & the Madness of Crowds,* published in England in 1841.[8] Already, in mid-nineteenth-century Europe, Mackay had plenty of examples of self-deception that rose to the level of a collective illusion, scams and follies that gripped large numbers of people and, sometimes, whole nations: the tulip mania in Holland, alchemy, the Great Crusades, and the witch burnings are just a few of those he cited. Every age is susceptible to its unique version of self-deceiving folly. Starting in the mid-twentieth century, one of ours was the outsize role attributed to the brain by psychiatry and society in determining all we think, feel, and do.

Psychiatry has always been viewed with some suspicion. One hears it said, sometimes in jest, sometimes seriously, that psychiatrists are more abnormal than the patients they treat (no one claims that cardiologists have worse hearts than their patients or that surgeons are themselves in need of surgery). Hollywood has often portrayed psychiatrists as betraying their patients, while simultaneously destroying themselves. Perhaps these filmmakers, and the writers who create the stories behind their films, are the ultimate seers into the human condition. Freud himself acknowledged, "Imaginative writers are valuable colleagues. In the knowledge of the human heart they are far ahead of us common folk."[9] Maybe these creative people knew all along that psychiatry never really did get it right, or serve its patients well, not when psychoanalysis was in vogue and certainly not now that biological psychiatry runs the show.[10]

The affront to psychiatry caused by the insistence that all mental illness derives from a brain chemical imbalance occurred simultaneously with a general decline in Western culture. People used to talk about "selling out," which meant giving up what they really believed in, usually for the promise of fame or money. Selling out once implied a lower level of personal integrity and satisfaction. These days, that lower level is unabashedly courted by most people from the start, and no one feels the less for beginning at that level, or staying there. The closest anyone comes now to acknowledging an ultimate good in the workplace is what the business world likes to call "creating value for shareholders." This is the program the drug companies follow as they continue to help define and bankroll biological psychiatry. What a fine way to say that greed is the only good, as the Michael Douglas character Gordon Gecko does in the iconic 1987 film *Wall Street*. In this new ethical dispensation, Gecko may make our skin crawl, but there is no contravening ethos strong enough to convince us that he is wrong, either.

It is no surprise that, in the absence of any other value, money filled the vacuum as the default value and became the ultimate desideratum. Many psychiatrists now are acquiescing to billable hours and the bottom line as the primary objectives of their work. I have colleagues who, at the end of the day, wonder if any goal other than survival is even worth considering. Freud understood that those under attack often identify with the aggressor as a strategy for dealing with their anxiety and surviving the onslaught. Simply put, psychiatrists have surrendered to market forces. Gratification delayed during years of medical and specialty training calls out to be slaked, school tuition and the mortgage need to be paid, and a dignified retirement must be secured.

A psychiatrist friend, who has spent his entire career on the staff of one of the country's premier psychiatric hospitals and is about to retire, told me with a hint of smugness that he made $200,000 during the previous year. Then he told me, without any detectable regret, that he was seeing over 400 patients a month. This is a clinician who started his career doing therapy with patients, then, under pressure, turned to doing three medication checks an hour. Some psychiatrists I know have started referring to themselves as neuropsychiatrists or psychopharmacologists to emphasize their allegiance to the currently fashionable—and profitable—quick fix. Others left the profession in disgust and despair.

As a clinician who writes about patients, I am imbued with what Albert Camus saw as the writer's responsibility to be a *witness* to the injustices of his time.[11] Staying silent after seeing people harmed by the ultimate "helping profession" would be to tacitly accept this dark irony. For the better part of a decade, though I was sometimes critical of how so many of the patients I worked with in the ER had been misdiagnosed and wrongly medicated, I did not directly question the integrity of the profession itself. The articles and the book, *Psych ER*, that I wrote based on this experience came mostly from inside the box. But then I gradually came to see that much of what made up psychiatry's "box" had indeed become toxic. From that point on, to be true to my patients and to myself, I would have to think, practice, and write somewhat outside the box.

CHAPTER 2
How Biological Psychiatry Lost the Mind and Went Brain Dead

In 1980, the American Psychiatric Association put out a new edition of the *Diagnostic and Statistical Manual of Mental Disorders*, its third. Spearheaded and edited by Robert L. Spitzer, the goal of the *DSM-III* was to create an "objective" psychiatry. This was to be a new paradigm that would set psychiatry on a firm scientific foundation.[1] In deliberately objectifying symptoms by ignoring their meaning, the plan was to save psychiatry from the "soft," subjective method of psychoanalysis that had informed the first two editions of the *DSM*. With this "hard," objective, and scientific stance, it was anticipated that psychiatry would become more like the other medical specialties.

The problem with this objective approach was that real life is *subjective* to the core. It is just this "soft," messy stuff in human experience that has to be acknowledged and assessed if the abnormal behavior that is labeled as a mental disorder can be understood and clinically challenged. When symptoms of unspecified meaning are used to make a diagnosis—*when the behavior itself is taken to be the illness, without regard for the part that behavior plays in the totality of the patient's life*—this subjective experience gets frozen out. Resorting to yet another metaphor, the essence of what is required to make a valid diagnosis lands on the cutting-room floor.

In *Brave New Brain*, Nancy C. Andreasen seemed pleased when she noted, "Since the development of the *DSM III* the entire process of defining mental illnesses and making diagnoses has become both objective and public."[2] To be objective in this way requires that pathological experience and behavior be reduced to symptoms that are taken at face value, without regard for the context or meaning of the behavior being assessed. Objectivity somehow became conflated with validity here, as psychiatry moved closer to medicine.

Even in somatic medicine, whose standards psychiatry hoped to adopt, symptoms are not always objective. No one who has witnessed repeated chest-pain-rule-out-MI evaluations in the emergency room would maintain that patients who come in with this kind of pain are having objective symptoms. Ultimately, the ER attending must determine what the pain reported by the patient signifies. Does it originate in the musculature of the chest, or in the skeleton, or does it come from under the sternum? Is it anginal, the result of restricted blood flow in the coronary arteries? Or worse, is it due to cell death in cardiac muscle caused by a shut-down of that flow?

An electrocardiogram and cardiac enzyme levels may or may not be helpful in establishing the meaning of the pain reported by the patient. Even when there is a physiological cause, symptoms can be subjective because they are being experienced and described by a person who is subjective. Finding the origin and the meaning of a patient's symptoms, and then making a valid diagnosis, involves the art of medicine as well as the practice of medical science.[3]

Delirium is known to have over 100 antecedents. Electrolyte and endocrine imbalances, as well as the ingestion of a number of toxic substances, are just a few of the conditions that can disrupt normal brain function to produce alterations in mental status. It is generally agreed that because of the medical illness exclusion criteria that were initiated with the *DSM-III* and continued in subsequent editions, the diagnosis of mental disorders due to medical and physiological conditions has been greatly improved. Many patients who present with psychiatric symptoms caused by these conditions are now being spared a wrong diagnosis of a primary mood disorder or a schizophrenia spectrum disorder. Several years before the publication of the *DSM-III* in1980, one of my friends, then in his mid-30s, was hospitalized for alcohol dependence and depression. In spite of having had the classic symptoms of alcoholic hallucinosis and no prior psychotic experiences, he was diagnosed with schizophrenia! It is less likely that this mistake would be made today.

If a clinician can tie a psychiatric symptom to a medical or physiological condition, the origin and meaning of that symptom are established. It is with primary mood disorders and schizophrenia spectrum disorders that do not have an obvious medical or physiological component that the *DSM*'s disregard for the meaning of symptoms has led to so much wrong diagnosis.[4,5]

In *Brave New Brain*, Andreasen acknowledged the limitations of diagnosing patients using objective, behavioral criteria, even as her enthusiasm for doing so was obvious. What she says here about schizophrenia is true also of bipolar disorder.

> When *DSM III* was written, however, concerns about overdiagnosis of schizophrenia and poor reliability led to an emphasis on symptoms that were easily defined because they were more objective than subjective. Specifically, the definition emphasized hallucinations (hearing voices) and delusions (a variety of false beliefs, such as being controlled by outside forces or persecuted). The definition of schizophrenia became more reliable with the new *DSM III* criteria, but the essence of its concept may have been lost in the process.[6]

Here is an acknowledgment that, in the *DSM-III* and its later revisions, subjectivity has yielded to objectivity and that validity (accurately naming a patient's pathological experience) has taken second place to reliability (allowing multiple clinicians to come up with the same diagnosis, right or wrong). Many clinicians now feel that as long as the makers of the *DSM* insist on trying to give us an objective psychiatry and continue to ignore the subjectivity that is the essence of both "normal" and pathological thinking, feeling, and behavior, we will persist in laboring under a classification and diagnostic system that often misses the point, and ultimately the patient.[7,8]

Though the *DSM-IV* is a compendium of mental disorders, nowhere in this volume that is thick with lists of psychiatric symptoms is the concept of mind ever defined. Nor is there any discussion of the role played by the mind in generating and sustaining mental disorders. In a section titled "Definition of a Mental Disorder," the following explanation is given for the dilemma faced by clinicians as they try to diagnose a mental disorder without a concept of mind.

> [T]he term *mental disorder* unfortunately implies a distinction between "mental" disorders and "physical" disorders that is a reductionistic anachronism of mind/body dualism. A compelling literature documents that there is much "physical" in "mental" disorders and much "mental" in "physical" disorders. The problem raised by the term "mental" disorders has been much clearer than its solution, and, unfortunately, the term persists in the title of DSM-IV because we have not found an appropriate substitute.[9]

This same nondefinition of a mental disorder appeared earlier, in exactly the same words, in both the *DSM-III* (1980) and the *DSM-III-R* (1987), and later in the *DSM-IV-TR* (2000). With all the progress psychiatry claims to have made in understanding and treating mental illness, the makers of the *DSM-IV* seem to be conceding that, in the two decades between 1980 and 2000, no progress was made in deciding what a mental disorder is, or, for that matter, what the mind is. I would offer this rudimentary definition: *the mind is the constituting power of consciousness, an active, ongoing, purposeful operation that involves free will, meaning, and choice, which is dependent for its functioning on an active, reciprocal brain substrate.*

That the lack of a concept of mind might impede psychiatry's efforts to parse the varieties of mental illness is not acknowledged in the *DSM-IV.* This omission signals that the mind, once considered to be the seat of all we think, feel, and do, is no longer seen in that way. In fact, a good deal of knowledge about the mind that psychiatry accumulated during the century before biological psychiatry became the dominant paradigm is given short shrift here. The *DSM-IV*'s silence on the role played by the mind in mental illness created a vacuum that was gradually filled by the empirical findings of a fast-developing brain science, though this result was not the intention of the authors of the *DSM-III.*

This next quote from the *DSM-IV* can be taken as further evidence that objective psychiatry tends to emphasize mental illness as an entity in itself at the expense of considering what has happened to the patient who is mentally ill.

> A common misconception is that a classification of mental disorders classifies people, when actually what are being classified are disorders that people have. For this reason, the text of *DSM-IV* (as did the text of *DSM-III-R*) avoids the use of such expressions as "a schizophrenic" or "an alcoholic" and instead uses the more accurate, but admittedly more cumbersome, "an individual with Schizophrenia" or "an individual with Alcohol Dependence."[10]

In choosing to classify mental disorders as something people *have*, rather than as something that is inseparable from who they *are*, the makers of the *DSM* attempted to distinguish the illness from the patient. To name a patient as "an individual *with* schizophrenia" (emphasis added), and to deny that he *is* a schizophrenic (possibly in a misguided bow to political correctness), is to put distance between the person and the illness, and to think of the illness as more objective than subjective. The essential distinction made here is an ontological one between *Being* and *Having.* (Ontology is the branch of philosophy concerned with Being.) Broadly, Being is what I *am*, Having is what I *have*. In the strictest sense of the term, I can only *have* something whose existence is external to me.

The Being/Having distinction bears the wound of Western, Cartesian thinking, dividing as it does some aspect of human experience into two parts. In his existentialist diary *Being and Having*, Gabriel Marcel recognized this dichotomy as false and tried to undercut it, even as he defined it.

> … I find myself confronted with things: and some of these things have a relationship with me which is at once peculiar and mysterious. These things are not *only external*: it is as though there were a connecting corridor between them and me; they reach me, one might say, underground. In exact proportion as I am attached to these things, they are seen to exercise a power over me which my attachment confers upon them, and which grows as the attachment grows. There is one particular thing which really stands first among them, or which enjoys an absolute priority, in this respect, over them—my body … It seems that my body literally devours me, and it is the same with all the other possessions which are somehow attached or hung upon my body.[11]

The more a person's body is affected by an illness the more that body comes to seem like a possession. When one feels well, the body is a part of the good feeling, and does not announce itself as something separate and distinct. But as soon as the body is overtaken by illness, particularly when there is pain and disability, the previously taken-for-granted body comes front and center, and begins to feel foreign, like something the patient *has*. But—and Marcel helps us see why—that illness cannot be separated from who the patient *is*, either. The *DSM-IV*, in the ultimate Cartesian reduction, ripped the person out of his natural world and transformed his illness into a *thing*, something he *has* that is *not him*, which needs to be studied as a thing and treated as a thing.

Ontologically, the patient "with schizophrenia" is also "a schizophrenic." In denying this reality, psychiatry lost what it used to think of as the mind, and the patient along with it. One does not have to look beyond this jettisoning of mind, so readily acknowledged in the *DSM-IV* as a deliberate effort to avoid a "reductionistic anachronism of mind/body dualism," to understand how the practice of psychiatry has taken root in an illusion. In what is surely one of the great ironies of Western thought, the *DSM*, in attempting to avoid a reduction to the mind, created instead what amounts to a reduction to the brain. While understanding someone's life as the product of a brain that lacks the capacity of an autonomous mind, a clinician cannot possibly know what the patient's life-story narrative means, what the symptoms extracted from the story mean, what the level of pathology (if any) is, and what the diagnosis might be, let alone what the treatment should be. In place of an understanding of what it means to be human, biological psychiatry has substituted the Holy Grail of a brain science that promises to explain mental illness, and cure it. As long as no one can prove that the Holy Grail does not exist, there is sufficient incentive for all invested parties to continue looking for it.

The illusion that biological psychiatry eventually became originated in the truth that the worst mental illnesses—correctly diagnosed schizophrenia and bipolar disorder—have roots in a disordered brain substrate. The illusion is one of extension, culminating in the claim that the biological provenance of these illnesses is the provenance of *all* pathological thinking, feeling, and behavior. In the early twentieth century, the German psychiatrist Eugen Bleuler chose the word *schizophrenia*, derived from the Greek, to signify that some of his sickest patients thought, felt, and behaved as if they had a "divided mind." In 1984, Nancy C. Andreasen, a contemporary American psychiatrist, titled a book *The Broken Brain: The Biological Revolution in Psychiatry.*[12] Like Bleuler, Andreasen saw mental illness as a compromise of the integrity, or wholeness, of the affected person. But she did not attribute the "brokenness" to the mind as Bleuler had done, or to an entity called the self, as R.D. Laing did in *The Divided Self,*[13] but to a compromised biological substrate. In biological psychiatry, mind and self are seen as broken because the brain is broken.

The downplaying of the mind that began with the publication of the *DSM-III* in 1980 was part of psychiatry's change in approach from a psychoanalytic and psychodynamic understanding of human behavior to one based on faulty brain function. From a developing, white-hot neuroscience, biological psychiatry inherited a vocabulary and syntax that replaced the vocabulary and syntax of psychoanalysis: conscious, unconscious, ego, superego, id, defense mechanism, neurosis, and psychosis were overtaken by neuron, neurotransmitter, synapse, synaptic cleft, presynaptic receptor, postsynaptic receptor, and reuptake receptor. The new language of brain science then made it possible to talk about a connection between something called a "chemical imbalance" and a mental disorder such as anxiety, depression, bipolar disorder, and schizophrenia, and to provide a rationale for prescribing drugs to correct the imbalance. Using this new vocabulary, most of the attention focused on how drugs bind to cell receptors (portals of access to cells that control the way cells function), as well as the signaling between neurons. It was posited that, by altering the structure and function of receptors in brain cells of neurons that modulate mood, cognition, and behavior, the abnormal neurotransmission presumed to underlie a mental disorder could be rectified. This is where the notion of the chemical imbalance comes from.[14]

No one who is familiar with the advances made in neuroscience and psychopharmacology during the last 50 years would deny that some patients, usually those who were the most seriously ill, were helped by drugs introduced during this time. But with that success came the idea that *every* mental illness had a biological cause, and that the mind was an epiphenomenon. Between psychiatry, the managed care companies, and Big Pharma (a term coined to name the economic and political clout of the pharmaceutical industry), a collective illusion took hold that relegated the mind to the slag heap, along with the capacities attributed to it: consciousness, freedom, choice, and the will to power.

An illusion of this magnitude and duration could not have begun, and would not have thrived, unless it filled the needs of a large number of people. Neuroscientists and biological psychiatrists got the satisfaction of feeling they had discovered a new truth about mental illness by connecting it to a "hard" science. They saw themselves as the "good guys" who showed up the "bad guys," those psychiatrists who had been influenced by psychoanalysis, which, they said, was mired in myth and had no validity. Big Pharma saw a chance to cash in, and funded research at universities and medical schools.[15] As the market for their products grew, these companies spent enormous amounts of money trying to convince doctors and the public that their drugs were the answer to the pain and inconvenience of anxiety, depression, mood swings, and psychosis.

This new way of doing psychiatry meant that managed care companies and health maintenance organizations (HMOs) could say good-bye to the days when a patient with a mental disorder was hospitalized for months, or sometimes years. Those who were paying the bill wanted psychiatrists to start medication immediately, reduce symptoms, and discharge the patient as soon as possible for outpatient follow-up. Faster, better, cheaper.

Hospitals and psychiatrists quickly recognized the wave of the future, and followed the money. President George H.W. Bush declared 1990 to 2000 to be the "Decade of the Brain." His Presidential Proclamation listed mental illness, along with Alzheimer's disease and Parkinson's disease, as brain diseases that would eventually be conquered by medical science. The federal government poured its resources into funding the biological psychiatry juggernaut.

Once biology had been posited as the cause of most mental illness, a confluence of forces energized by this idea virtually guaranteed that psychiatry would betray itself and its patients. A giant blind spot caused by the ablated mind made it all but impossible for a psychiatrist to understand and confront what was really happening when a patient came for help with a problem. Frustration, dissatisfaction, unhappiness, guilt, anger, and even feelings of inadequacy, which collectively account for most of what is being diagnosed as mental illness now, were reconceived as medical problems.[16] This change in perspective about what mental illness was reduced a person's complex life experience to a glitch in brain function that required correction with a drug.

A great deal is being said these days about why it is important for someone who is going into medicine, whatever the specialty, to seriously study the humanities. Medical schools are trying to break the traditional lock-step curriculum of college premed studies, which has emphasized science and rote memorization. Students interested in medical careers are being encouraged by colleges, and even medical schools, to take full majors in subjects like English, history, and psychology, while fulfilling premed requirements in biology, chemistry, and physics.

In spite of this trend, most psychiatrists are not well educated. Their training in medical school and residency does not encourage them to discover the surfaces, contours, and textures of the wider world. In fact, a grueling schedule tends to discourage them from doing so. Psychiatry, even as practiced at the highest level, is just one perspective on the world. The humanities, especially philosophy, psychology, literature, linguistics, and anthropology offer complementary views, allowing clinicians to see more deeply into the dysfunction and suffering of their patients. Psychiatrists need to have a sophisticated understanding of "normal" life so they can develop a context and a reference point for recognizing the pathological distortions in their patients' lives, and meet them in their disturbed world.

In *A Scream Goes Through the House*, subtitled *What Literature Teaches Us About Life*, Arnold Weinstein, a professor of comparative literature at Brown University, took on the question of how lives can be made better when people embrace the major texts in the Western literary canon. His work is in the tradition of the liberal arts, now devalued by a culture that is focused on technology and money-making. The liberal arts were intended to introduce a person to the world by teaching him to read, write, and think at a high level so he could live there more authentically and more freely.[17] Weinstein saw literature and art as a kind of antidote to what he calls the "shrinkage" in our lives, which is due to the limitations of the human condition itself, and to the compounding of these limitations by the life-denying ethos of our own time.

> [L]iterature and art *expand* our estate, enable us to move—conceptually, imaginatively, vicariously—out of the physical jail we (we the healthy, as well as we the sick) live in. This is not a cheat or an illusion. It is as real as the flesh that hurts, or even the death that is coming. The experience of art sets the brain and the heart going; it vitalizes and it quickens. I have argued, indeed, that it socializes and empowers, because it bids us to redefine "home" for us: art from other lands and times comes into us and enriches our estate; we move outward, into

> new territories that become ours. By offering us its special mirror, by showing how resonant and capacious the human story can be, art restores feeling to its proper place in life.[18]

To know what is pathological one must first know what is normal (a relative notion, to be sure), and getting to know the normal world is what studying the liberal arts helps us to do. I have learned as much about mental illness from a close reading of existential philosophy, novels, plays, poems, literary criticism, and from watching certain films as I have from reading the iconic texts of psychiatry and psychoanalysis. Just how one benefits from this kind of reading is hard to pin down. In his poem "Asphodel, That Greeny Flower," William Carlos Williams acknowledged how ineffable the lessons of literature can seem: "It is difficult / to get the news from poems / yet men die miserably every day / for lack / of what is found there."[19] A few simple words that appear to have been passed through a concentrating prism bring an announcement so powerful that it divides our world into the parts before and after we understood what Williams was saying.

Novelist Zoe Heller helps us to parse the "utility" of fiction when she reminds us that "literature cannot give absolute answers, or furnish watertight explanations. What it can do … is capture the moral tangle of personal life and historical context that is our lived experience."[20] Many psychiatric patients have problems that, ultimately, involve a "moral tangle" that is set in some "historical context," which is partly of their own making, and partly due to circumstance. The perspective here is distant enough to grasp the complexities of meaning and structure underlying someone's mental illness, and close enough to consider the "lived experience" of the suffering person.

Psychiatrists who do not have such an encompassing perspective, however this is achieved, work from a deficit, one that will not be disclosed by examinations taken in medical school and residency training, or for board certification. They will not be able to understand psychopathological theory, how to identify and diagnosis a mental illness from the stories patients tell, or how to take a therapeutic stand against an illness. I am convinced that this deficit is one of the reasons many psychiatrists, in spite of their excellent credentials, do not help their patients, and sometimes harm them.

Biological psychiatrists have not only ignored what can be learned from the liberal arts, they have often rejected the psychoanalytic, psychodynamic, and existential theories of the mind that were developed, refined, and tested in clinical practice during the last century. This work has been dismissed as unscientific, and replaced by theories of the brain based on neuroscience and psychopharmacology.

In spite of the emphasis traditionally put on the study of physical and biological science in medical school, psychiatrists are really not all that well trained in science, either. Most importantly, they are not equipped to evaluate the work of those scientists who generate empirical data that are used to posit a connection between some abnormal brain function and a mental disorder. The leap made from the hard science of laboratory measurements—including supposed determinations of neurotransmitter levels and real-time visualizations of brain function on the color-coded monitors of brain scanners—to the abnormal productions of consciousness is a stretch of dubious validity. In these measurements, some mental disorder is related to some marker that is related to some molecular function in some part of the brain that has been shown to be associated with feeling, thinking, and behavior. The *association* is then promoted as an *explanation* for the illness, with the implication that the illness is now *understood.* A blurring of epistemological terms is at the heart of the illusion that every mental illness is a brain illness. Giving his take on MTV, Pete Townsend, the guitarist and primary songwriter for The Who from 1964 to 1982, said: "You can speak a language there where nothing you say needs to make sense, but everyone understands you anyway."[21] This is how it is in much of the discourse that drives the illusion of biological psychiatry.

When medicine, business, the federal government, and society made the brain, rather than the mind, the major target in the effort to understand and treat mental illness, most psychiatrists bought the illusion hook, line, and sinker. Undoubtedly, an important, subconscious factor here was the pull of self-deception.[22] As the journalist Upton Sinclair recognized, "It's difficult to get a man to understand something when his salary depends on his not understanding it."[23]

A quasi-religious fervor marks the commitment of many people who are caught up in the collective illusion of biological psychiatry. It is *presumed* now that science should be the arbiter of everything significant about mental illness. It is *presumed* that science will come up with "cures"—or at least palliative strategies—for the disorders in the *DSM-IV.*

Rollo May, a psychologist whose perspective on the world was influenced by existential philosophy, challenged these presumptions.

> In our day of dedication to facts and hard-headed objectivity, we have disparaged imagination: it gets us away from "reality"; it taints our work with "subjectivity"; and, worst of all, it is said to be unscientific. As a result, art and imagination are taken as the "frosting" to life rather than as the solid food.
>
> What if imagination and art are not frosting at all, but the fountainhead of human experience? What if our logic and our

> science derive from art forms and are fundamentally dependent on them …?[24]

May is claiming that art—and this includes the liberal arts—trumps science as the way to pursue the ultimate meaning of human experience.

Contrary to what the makers of the *DSM-IV* say, having a concept of mind is compatible with the seemingly indisputable fact that some brain function underlies every thought, emotion, and act. In this sense, everything is biological. There would be no mind, no imagination, no subjectivity, and no consciousness without a functioning brain substrate, as we know from observing the consequences of trauma, dementia, and other insults to the brain. But, in spite of what biological psychiatry and the drug companies would have us believe, the data derived from a large and growing literature do not explain the essence of *any* mental illness. We simply do not know how the productions of consciousness are derived from the workings of the brain.

CHAPTER 3

The Brain Cannot Account for What We Think, Feel, and Do

Near the end of *Listening to Prozac*, Peter Kramer all but acknowledged the death of the mind for psychiatry: "A few decades after he proposed it, Sartre's notion of nausea as the most basic of human emotions is dismissed by most psychologists and philosophers."[1] Kramer did well to look to Jean-Paul Sartre for a model of the mind, even though it is one based as much on emotion as on cognition.

Published in 1938, Sartre's novel *Nausea* told the story of the young Frenchman, Antoine Roquentin, who comes to know and to feel what it means, in the parlance of existential philosophy, *to exist*. But before that can happen, he has to pull himself out of the deep malaise he has fallen into while writing a book about an obscure French nobleman. During that time, Roquentin had no life, as people like to say now. Most of his hours were spent absorbed in and distracted by every detail of the life of a man long dead, his literary quarry. For Roquentin, this quest amounted to a roundabout, self-deceiving effort *not to exist*. Eventually, his inauthentic life became so dysfunctional that he no longer felt real, and he was unable to continue working on the book. What Roquentin did feel during the time when he was lost to himself was *nausea*—the somatic sensation Sartre associates with self-deception. Roquentin is Sartre's poster boy for the inauthentic life.

Then, one day, while sitting on a park bench and staring at the root of a chestnut tree, Roquentin has an intuition that changes his life.

> *I exist*, I am the one who keeps it up. I. The body lives by itself once it has begun. But thought—*I* am the one who continues it, unrolls it. I exist ....
>
> My thought is *me*. I exist because I think ... and I can't stop myself from thinking .... *I am the one* who pulls myself from the nothingness to which I aspire ...[2]

Sartre convinces us that Roquentin has turned a corner, and started living his own life. He grasps his *contingency*, the cold, hard fact that it is *he* who will determine the person he becomes ("I exist because I think."). Once Roquentin stops deceiving himself about what it means to live, his body comes alive as well: he feels the saliva in his mouth, the warmth of his skin, his weight on the floor. Sartre tells us that before he embraced his contingency and became an active player in his life, Roquentin had been so passive that the objects he encountered seemed to *touch him*. Even after grasping his contingency, Roquentin acknowledges an inclination to backslide into the nothingness and the nausea he so recently overcame. The challenge to be authentic—"to exist"—is ongoing.

Today, people who experience the equivalent of Roquentin's nausea—feeling anxious, depressed, bored, or empty—are told that the problem is not in their mind, as Roquentin came to realize about himself, but in their brain. In this way of looking at what it means to be human, the axis of contingency no longer turns on acts of will underwritten by the mind, but on what is going on in neural networks that modulate mood, deep in the brain.

Sartre, and those who think like him, insist that Roquentin's discovery that his life is contingent on how he constitutes his experience moment to moment ("*I* am the one who continues it") is a fact of life for everyone, whether this is acknowledged or not. Perhaps the doubters will be persuaded by the following story, which is just one of an infinite number of stories that could be told to support the idea of contingency.[3] It is commencement day at a Midwestern university. A young woman (let's call her Alex) is waiting for her boyfriend (let's call him John), who had graduated the previous year, to come from a distant city for the ceremony. A friend tells Alex that her roommate, who is also due to graduate that day, had been sleeping with John when he was still a student, while Alex believed they had an exclusive relationship. Calling from his car, John announced that he would arrive shortly. Speaking from her dorm room, Alex announced that John should turn his car around and never contact her again.

We do not know how long it took Alex to process the news about John's betrayal, but it probably did not take long. In a short time, Alex's view of John, which had been sufficiently positive for her to sustain a relationship with him for two years, changed so drastically that she forever exiled him from her life. Would those who claim that we are no more than what our brain is doing at any moment ask us to believe that Alex's brain autonomously changed its neural tone in the circuits underlying her feelings for him? Or would it be more reasonable to posit that her positive feelings—contingent on the presumption that John was good, decent, loyal—could no longer be sustained, and that she could now feel only loathing? Did Alex's *brain* "decide" to blow this guy off, or did *she* make that call?

Anger, anxiety, and humiliation must have been some of the components of Alex's experience, and her brain must have responded to the bad news with an alteration in neural function and tone. But it was the constituting power of Alex's mind that initiated these changes in brain activity—a mind that had given one meaning to her relationship with John before she knew of his betrayal, then a diametrically opposite meaning after she discovered it.

Biological psychiatry denies this very same mind an autonomous role in creating and sustaining a mental illness. That the mind eventually would be replaced by the functioning brain was a consequence of a trend in Western thought that started with Plato and Aristotle and reached its apex during the Enlightenment with the work of the French philosopher René Descartes (1596–1650), who famously declared "I think, therefore I am." The split implied here between mind and world, or, more specifically, between thinking and everything else people do, had already been a staple in the analytical philosophy of the Greeks who followed Socrates, as well as in the natural science that came later, long before Descartes wrote the words that were destined to be carved in stone.

The *Cogito*, as it is commonly known, became iconic because Descartes, with the simple words "I think, therefore I am," identified the way philosophers and scientists had been thinking at that time, and continue to think now. Descartes did not originate the split between mind and world,[4] though the approach he took in his own philosophizing greatly helped to perpetuate it. The ultimate meaning of the *Cogito* is that Descartes turned his back on the complex and messy world that people live in—one filled with doubt and the anxiety that inheres in doubt—and constructed in his mind a series of meditations about this world that systematically reduced doubt. (It was Descartes's reduction of the doubt-ridden world to an idealized facsimile that, starting 300 years later, the existentialists revolted against. They maintained that philosophical thinking should engage life directly, without splitting the thinking mind from the reality of uncertainty.)

Once the tie between person and world was broken by the *Cogito*, it was only a matter of time before enough information accumulated about the structure and function of the two-pound mass of cells and electrical circuits known as the brain for *it* to be posited as the essence of what makes us human. "I think, therefore I am" became "I have a brain, therefore I am." Biological psychiatry's morphing of mind to brain must be counted as one of the great ironies in Western intellectual history: the mind discovered and characterized the brain, only to be displaced by it as the essence of life.

Francis Crick, a British molecular biologist who shared the Nobel Prize with James Watson in 1962 for their discovery of the double helical structure of DNA, later turned his attention to exploring how the brain works in shaping human consciousness. Crick opened his 1994 book *The Astonishing Hypothesis* with this salvo: "The Astonishing Hypothesis is that 'You,' your joys and your sorrows, your memories and your ambitions, your sense of personal identity and free will, are in fact no more than the behavior of a vast assembly of nerve cells and their associated molecules ... You're nothing but a pack of neurons."[5]

Francis Crick was a theoretician, not a clinician, and he never worked with patients. Nancy C. Andreasen is the Andrew H. Woods Chair of Psychiatry at The University of Iowa College of Medicine and was editor-in-chief of *The American Journal of Psychiatry* from 1992 to 2005. She is a clinician, and has based most of her large body of published work on studies with patients who had psychiatric disorders. In *Brave New Brain: Conquering Mental Illness in the Era of the Genome*, which came out in 2001, she discusses her own research and presents the bona fides of biological psychiatry, tracing the paradigm shift from a mind-based psychoanalytic and psychodynamic perspective on mental illness to one emphasizing abnormal brain function. "The brain," Andreasen tells us, "forms the essence of what defines us as human beings. To understand its structure and its workings is to understand ourselves."[6] Francis Crick would agree entirely. This is the intellectual soil that nourished biological psychiatry.

To buttress her argument that mental illness is a brain illness, Andreasen tries to convince us that some well-known medical illnesses—including Huntington's disease, Parkinson's disease, Alzheimer's disease, and syphilis—are *mental illnesses*! To be sure, these brain diseases significantly affect mental status, causing depression, psychosis, and dementia, particularly in the latter stages of the illness. But Andreasen asks us to believe that these neurological disorders are "mental illnesses" in the same way that anxiety, depression, bipolar disorder, and schizophrenia are mental illnesses. This kind of thinking starts us sliding down a slippery slope, blurring distinctions that must be maintained if we are to learn more about why people are anxious, depressed, have severe mood swings, and lose contact with reality.[7] Brain diseases with psychiatric sequelae, such as Huntington's, Parkinson's, Alzheimer's, and syphilis, have a known neurological substrate. Illnesses that can be thought of as primary mental illnesses do not, as Andreasen acknowledges.

> As the tools and methods of molecular genetics and molecular biology became steadily more refined during the late 1970s and early 1980s, investigators had high hopes that they could be used rapidly to identify disease mechanisms for a variety of major illnesses .... The gene for Huntington's disease was identified quickly, causing many to believe that other mental illnesses would be equally easy ...[8]

That was not the case. Andreasen explains, "With the exception of Huntington's disease, for which a dominant and fully penetrant gene has been found, we have no definitive markers or diagnostic tests for any mental illness that can be administered to living people."[9] But still she insists that mental illness is biologically determined, and that the mind does not play a major role in its development. "Most of the factors that produce a 'broken brain' are outside the control of the individual who develops the illness, although he or she does have 'free will' in deciding how to cope with its consequences."[10]

Andreasen's take on "free will" would seem to account for the limiting situation faced by those who are compromised by the neurological disorders that she wants us to believe are also mental illnesses. But she misses how those spared from this kind of neurological impairment might respond inadequately and inauthentically to the circumstances of life in such a way as to produce anxiety or depression, mood swings, and even distortions of cognition and perception. If the "broken brain" is the cause of a mental illness and "most factors" that "produce" this condition are "outside the control of the individual who develops the illness," as Andreasen claims, a mindless individual is at the mercy of his brain when things start to go badly, and his only response is to "cope with [the] consequences." Not *reverse* the consequences, mind you, just "cope" with them. It follows that, if the individual had nothing to do with creating his illness in the first place, there is no a priori reason to expect that he can do anything to change the situation once he becomes ill.

Andreasen would deny Roquentin the power of his epiphany—the realization that it is *he* who determines his life, and he who ultimately determines whether he will feel the nausea that accompanies a self-deceiving and self-diminishing approach to it. According to her, the "broken brain" cannot mobilize the mind's power of will to respond authentically to life. (We are never told why or how a brain "breaks" in the first place—this is a metaphor that lacks a literal reference point.)

Any attempt to explain mental illness implicitly requires a reciprocal concept of "normal" human experience, which could be defined somewhat tautologically as the absence of debilitating pathology. "If mind and brain are different facets of the same thing," Andreasen asks, "where is the moral executor? Where is personal identity and the chance to make choices about what we might do or become? If we are the product of the activity of our brains, then where and who are WE?"[11] These are ultimate questions that cut to the heart of life, philosophy, and biological psychiatry, and are put in stark terms. Andreasen's answers are no less stark. She feels that, collectively, these matters are "philosophical or religious ... rather ... than scientific ... for which we are unlikely to demonstrate a neural basis or mechanism."[12]

Here we have the exposed bare bones of biological psychiatry: In reducing all we are to our brain, the rest of what we are is simply not psychiatry's business. "Mother Theresa will teach us more about the soul than a PET scan can,"[13] Andreasen assures us, with a touch of hauteur, clearly ridding psychiatry of the obligation. She comes to essentially the same conclusion about the mind as did the makers of the *DSM-IV*. With a similar sleight of hand, they also declined to take responsibility for defining what is "mental" about a mental disorder, pleading that doing so would amount to a "reductionistic anachronism of mind/body dualism."[14] Refusing to reduce a human being to his mind, Andreasen and the *DSM* proudly reduce him to his brain. This is how the mind was lost for psychiatry.

Perhaps the way to show that we are more than the sum of our neural firings would be to live *as if* we were free, rather than by trying to prove the point through a logical argument. In a letter to a young friend, the German poet Rainer Maria Rilke (1875–1926) gave this advice: "Don't search for the answers ... because you would not be able to live them. And the point is, to live everything. *Live* the questions now. Perhaps then, someday far in the future, you will gradually, without even noticing it, live your way into the answer."[15] Rilke's Zen-like words point us toward the kind of engagement with the world that our Western, dualistic consciousness often precludes. One way into that world is through the mind, which is why it was such a terrible thing for psychiatry to lose.

CHAPTER 4

The Lost Art of Psychiatric Diagnosis

When psychiatry lost the mind, it also lost its hold on psychiatric diagnosis. Like so many medical terms, *diagnosis* has its roots in the Greek. *Stedman's Medical Dictionary* defines *gnosia* as "The perceptive faculty enabling one to recognize the form and nature of persons and things; the faculty of perceiving and recognizing."[1] *Dia* means through or completely. To diagnose is to see through and to know something completely—to know its *meaning*.

In claiming that the mind and its workings are nothing more than the action of the brain, biological psychiatry leveraged what is essentially a crude understanding of neural processes into a theory of brain function that purports to explain both normal and abnormal behavior. Giving this much power to the brain was a revolution in Western thought and made people see themselves in a different way. If neural function is the most important determinant of what makes us who we are, then we—our selves—are no longer thinking, feeling, and acting with a free will that implies meaning. If normal behavior has no meaning, then neither does abnormal behavior, and what psychiatry calls symptoms are "meaningless," too.

Looking back at the history of the *DSM*, the makers of the *DSM-IV* acknowledged the excision of meaning from their new codification of mental illness: "*DSM-III* introduced a number of important methodological innovations, including explicit diagnostic criteria, a multiaxial system, and *a descriptive approach that attempted to be neutral with respect to theories of etiology*."[2] (italics added) These "theories of etiology" were, for the most part, psychoanalytic theories of the mind. The diagnostic schemas of the

DSM-II were constructed to capture a patient's subjectivity. But starting with the *DSM-III*, the intent to give the subjective its due morphed into an attempt to be objective by basing diagnosis on observed behavior.

Contrary to what most clinicians believe, the *DSM-III* and the *DSM-IV* were not intended primarily for diagnosing and treating mentally ill patients. Instead, these volumes were meant to accommodate the needs of those who do psychiatric research. Behavior, with no specified provenance or specified meaning, was chosen as the portal of access to mental illness because it was felt that behavior could be diagnosed reproducibly, or reliably, by multiple observers. The idea was that clinicians would all see the same behavior and make the same diagnosis. But the quest for reliability came at a price: the complex and messy subjective experience of a mentally ill patient had to be reduced to descriptions of aberrant and maladaptive behavior, and ultimately to a checklist of symptoms.

In guiding clinicians toward a diagnosis, the *DSM-III* and *DSM-IV* failed to take into account the meaning of what was happening in a patient's life. Reciprocally, inevitably, research based on the *DSM*'s meaningless diagnostic categories also fails to reflect a patient's lived reality. What good, we might ask, is research that bypasses the meaning of a mental illness? How could the results of such work benefit patients? The only obvious beneficiaries are the researchers themselves, who build careers on the results they publish.

Ironically, the plan to achieve objectivity and reliability in diagnosing mental disorders by using behavioral criteria did not work well. Without the possibility of considering what a patient's symptoms mean, different clinicians invariably ascribe *different* meanings to these symptoms. The belief that the *DSM-IV* promotes reliable diagnosis is increasingly being recognized as a myth.[3]

The psychoanalytically informed *DSM-II* was grounded in the idea that mental illness is caused by *internal conflicts* of the psyche. Hence the term psychodynamics, which names the psychic forces created by these conflicts. Conflicts, which Freud felt led to neurosis, have an implicit meaning because, if there were no meaning underlying human interaction, there would be nothing to be conflicted about. The *DSM-III* threw out conflict theory and made symptoms—which, unlike conflicts, could be observed rather than inferred—the criteria for diagnosis. The result came to be known as descriptive psychiatry, or phenomenology.

This phenomenology is not the existential phenomenology that informs the approach and method of philosophers such as Martin Heidegger, Jean-Paul Sartre, and Gabriel Marcel.[4] In their perspective on the world, and on mental illness, all human experience has meaning and structure, which can be studied and described. The *DSM-IV* "phenomenology" excludes meaning, hoping "to be neutral with respect to theories of etiology." In neutralizing etiology, the meaning of the observed symptoms was neutralized as well. No doubt, clinicians' attempts to diagnose meaningless symptoms were behind the numerous wrong diagnoses I encountered during the decade when I evaluated over 3,000 psychiatric patients in the emergency room.

Robert L. Spitzer, a professor of psychiatry at the Columbia College of Physicians and Surgeons, was the chief editor of the *DSM-III,* and its driving force.[5] Trained as a psychoanalyst as well as a psychiatrist, Spitzer became disillusioned with the analytic approach to understanding and treating mental illness. Spitzer never intended to deny the autonomy of the mind as he attempted to create an objective, descriptive psychiatry. That happened almost incidentally because, while the *DSM* was moving from an analytic to a descriptive ethos, another contingent in psychiatry was intent on establishing the brain as the principal determinant of behavior. Biological psychiatry implicitly adapted the "phenomenology" of the *DSM* to its own agenda by proposing a direct association between an observed abnormal behavior and a specific brain malfunction. In no case was the empirical evidence used to back up these claims sufficient to establish the association as a *cause* of the illness. Nonetheless, clinicians, researchers, pharmaceutical companies, and eventually patients themselves proceeded *as if* this cause had been established.

Emphasizing symptoms based on behavior and eschewing any probative theory to explain these symptoms, the *DSM-III* and its subsequent editions became the public face of psychiatry. These texts have often been dubbed the "bible" of mental illness. Worldwide sales made millions of dollars for the American Psychiatric Association. Clinicians found the *DSM-III* and its later revisions to be user-friendly and adopted this manual hook, line, and sinker for doing psychiatric diagnosis.

The attempt by the committee that gave us the *DSM-III* to create an "objective" psychiatry by objectifying human experience—which is constitutionally subjective to the core—may be one of the most misguided ideas in the history of Western thought. By definition, an objective symptom is a symptom whose meaning has been deliberately ignored—in a person whose very existence is meaningful! The "objective," behavioral symptoms used to establish the criteria for the diagnosis of mental disorders are often not valid because the subjective (meaningful) experience of the patients assessed has not been tapped into. In turn, results from research studies based on these "objective" criteria are used to determine the standard of care for clinical treatment. Invalid diagnostic criteria lead ineluctably to invalid patient care. This is all fruit from the poisoned tree of objectivity. (What can be labeled objective seems to be more "true" than what is merely subjective. A claim to objectivity brings psychiatry closer to the magisterium of medicine, which has roots in hard science.)

With the *DSM-III* came the concept of comorbidity,[6] which could have only originated in a diagnostic system based on meaningless symptoms. Comorbidity comes into play when a patient's symptoms fulfill the criteria for more than one *DSM* mental disorder. For example, depression may be a patient's most pressing problem. But the patient may also be anxious, have mood changes, display some obsessive-compulsive behavior, have lost control of his food intake, abuse drugs or alcohol. Instead of attempting to understand the patient's disordered behavior as a fundamental perturbation of what the German existential philosopher Martin Heidegger (1889–1976) called his *worlded Being*[7]—where each symptom represents a facet of the person's separation from the natural world and from others—the comorbidity of meaningless symptoms encourages a clinician to declare that distinct mental illnesses are at work, with each illness requiring a different medication. True, I am describing a worst-case scenario here. Yet this is how psychiatric diagnosis is often done now, and how treatment is initiated.

Reading what the British literary critic Clive James wrote about how he felt the poetry of Robert Lowell was constructed, it occurred to me that this, too, could be said of the way most *DSM* diagnoses are made: "Lowell thinks he is chipping away the marble to get at the statue. It's more likely that he is trying to build a statue out of marble chips."[8] A psychiatric diagnosis made with meaningless symptoms, especially when comorbidity is invoked, cannot render an accurate representation of a patient's troubled life. Instead, something reconstructed from a pile of "chips" is mistaken for a "statue." To make a correct diagnosis, the link between a patient and his world must be preserved so his story can reveal the elements of pathology that comprise the illness.

I offer the following cautionary tale to demonstrate how easy it is to be fooled while making a diagnosis when you do not know the patient's whole story and *do not realize that you do not know the whole story.*[9] A friend confided to me that the behavior of his son was causing him some concern. Art, who was in his mid-twenties, was acting out of character. He appeared anxious and confused, and was having more trouble than usual dealing with people. A college graduate, Art had quit a job selling subscriptions for a cable-television company and was supporting himself by delivering pizza. He seemed obsessed with his appearance, focusing painfully on features that he felt were unattractive. Art was particularly concerned about his body hair, which he was gradually having removed by an electrologist.

Art's father was a Rock of Gibraltar: solid, stable, dependable, giving, forgiving. His wife, Art's mother, on the other hand, lacked many of these qualities. A talented and published poet, she was emotionally brittle. She was frail, and at times looked spectral. Her emotional lability took its toll on both Art and his older married sister. Art seemed to favor his mother, while his sister had the father's emotional constitution.

At the very least, Art's mother appeared to be schizotypal. In her poetry, she acknowledged having had experiences that could be considered psychotic, though as far as I know she had never been diagnosed with or treated for any mental disorder. No doubt, this was due in part to the support of her husband, who worshiped his wife and championed her poetry. I often wondered how Art's mother would have fared had she not had this particular life partner. It seemed likely that it was his constant healing presence that kept her from decompensating into frank mental illness.

My friend asked for my advice about his son. The combination of Art's strange behavior and his mother's lifetime pattern of schizoptypal behavior made me wonder if Art was in the grip of some schizophrenia spectrum disorder (he had never abused drugs or alcohol). I referred him to a psychiatrist I knew and trusted. He declined to make the diagnosis I feared and prescribed a benzodiazepine for anxiety, but no other medication.

I did not hear anything about Art for almost a year. When I saw his father again he told me that Art had had sexual reassignment surgery; he was taking hormones and living as a woman. Art had kept his job delivering pizza and appeared to be doing well. As expected, the course he chose was not smooth, for either him or his father. Somehow, this young man had found a way to understand and then publicly acknowledge the feelings behind the behavior that had at first appeared so puzzling.

Many psychiatrists would have started Art on the road to being a schizophrenic patient. Art was fortunate, though his salvation from misdiagnosis did not lack irony. Adam, whose story follows, was not so fortunate.

CHAPTER 5

A Blatant Misdiagnosis of Schizophrenia

While making a sandwich for a customer, Adam cut his hand with a knife. The cut was not deep, did not bleed much, and did not need sutures. He stood back from the counter, overwhelmed by what had just happened. He felt anxious, and could not catch his breath. The casual conversation of the patient customers standing in front of the long deli case rose in his ears to a frightening pitch, though none of what he heard was in any way critical of him.

Adam's already tenuous identity began to crumble. He was no longer the eight-year employee of an upscale market who made sandwiches and filled gourmet orders to go. In the second it took to cut his hand, his familiar environment turned strange and hostile. Adam could no longer stay in the place where his identity had deserted him. He told his supervisor he needed to take the rest of the day off, and fled the store.

Adam drove back to his apartment. He called his psychiatrist, his drug counselor, his sister, his girlfriend, and me, his friend. Reaching out, he hoped to reconstitute his shattered sense of self and world, which was brittle even on his best days. His first words were, "I've just had another episode." Frightened and stunned by what had happened, he spoke fast, and was hyperventilating. But he was rational; he knew he had overreacted, and felt bad about it. His girlfriend said she would stop by later in the afternoon. His sister promised to come over after work.

Adam knew that almost anyone else would have been able to handle the trivial injury that had paralyzed and humiliated him. Not being able to take the ordinary in stride was Adam's hallmark. When he was 19, this flaw led to a life-altering event. Adam was struggling through his freshman year in college. During a lacrosse practice, when he was not performing well, the coach became annoyed. Words were exchanged, and there was pushing and shoving. The coach forced Adam to the ground. Then Adam got to his feet and pushed the coach to the ground. That night, the captain of the lacrosse team came to Adam's dorm room and told him that the coach was angry and was planning to "take Adam's head off." Adam panicked, taking the coach's threat to decapitate him at face value. He called his sister, who immediately came to the campus to bring him home. During the drive home, he drank a six-pack of beer.

Adam was failing most of his classes and reeling from a broken relationship with a woman he had been seriously involved with since high school. And, as Adam later told the dean of students, he had been "taking drugs non-stop" since he started college—large amounts of alcohol, marijuana, pills of all types, and LSD. He had used LSD the night before the incident with the coach.

Adam was admitted to a psychiatric hospital the next day, and four more times during the next five years. During one hospitalization, he was simultaneously on 11 psychotropic medications, including the neuroleptics Navane, Stelazine, and Thorazine. For 16 years, the most prominent feature of his psychiatric illness was a paranoia that was intractable to virtually every neuroleptic, atypical antipsychotic, mood stabilizer, anxiolytic, and antidepressant on the market. In spite of all this medication, Adam continued to be anxious, depressed, and paranoid and to have frequent panic attacks.

At age 35, Adam does not have the maturity and discriminatory power of an adult. In many ways he thinks, feels, and behaves like a child. He has episodes of enuresis, for which he takes Vivactil. Even on his best days he is unusually thin-skinned. Adam has histrionic and hypochondriacal traits. Hardly a waking hour goes by that he is not focusing on some aspect of his troubled psyche or aching body.

Adam is from an upper-middle-class WASP family, and went to private school. He retains his gentility, but is unable to keep up with the friends he made before becoming ill. A high school classmate, who had made millions in his own business, stopped by the store one day and flashed a $15,000 Rolex watch. Adam was being paid $9 an hour to make sandwiches behind a deli counter.

Since he was first hospitalized, Adam's diagnosis has been changed from schizophrenia to bipolar disorder to schizoaffective disorder. I have seen his mood swing from moderate, paranoid-flavored depression to brittle, false optimism, but I have never seen him manic, or even hypomanic. When he was told he had schizophrenia he did not challenge his doctors, but he did not believe them, either.

All through high school and for years after that, Adam drank alcohol heavily and, as he put it, used "every drug I could find." At the time he cut his hand, he had achieved some degree of control over his various addictions, but still used alcohol, marijuana, stimulants, and other drugs more often than he acknowledged to his psychiatrist, drug counselor, parents, and employer.

Adam's illness was rooted in anxiety and paranoia. After one paranoid episode that was precipitated by an unexplained noise in his apartment, I asked him if, in retrospect, he believed that any of his paranoid thoughts or feelings ever represented a real threat. Never, he said, unequivocally. That understanding, however, did nothing to forestall the next paranoid episode.

Adam's current psychiatrist told him that his symptoms do not squarely fit the *DSM-IV* criteria for schizophrenia, bipolar disorder, or schizoaffective disorder. Nonetheless, he provisionally diagnosed Adam with schizoaffective disorder, and medicated him for it. Adam denies ever having heard voices or having visual hallucinations, and I have not seen evidence of formal thought disorder. Adam sometimes feels that his coworkers at the store where he works are paying special attention to him, criticizing him behind his back and plotting against him. When he told me he feared that several men in the meat department might be planning to cut him up into pieces in the parking lot I asked myself if this fantasy, transient as it was, could be part of an actual delusional system. Most of Adam's paranoid episodes have the content and feel of extreme anxiety and panic.

At the time Adam cut his hand he was taking Prolixin, Depakote, Paxil, Wellbutrin, Inderal, and Akineton. Several atypical antipsychotics were also tried, but were less effective. Taking Prolixin, Adam was able to stay out of the hospital and struggle with the demands of making sandwiches behind a deli counter, all the time worrying that the customers and his coworkers were, in some unspecified way, against him. Adam startled me when he said he believed Prolixin worked for him because he focused on the *Pro* in the drug's name, which signified something positive that would take him forward. He also believes that Wellbutrin will make him well.

From the way Adam talks about the medication he takes now, it seems that, whatever effect these drugs are having on his brain, he also depends on them psychologically to control his mood and behavior. Perhaps this medication gives him a reason for functioning that he has not found elsewhere. He has done poorly when his medication was reduced or withdrawn. Adam often talks as if he needs drugs to regulate and integrate his life—prescription drugs now, along with the illicit ones he uses sporadically.

Adam started smoking cigarettes in high school, and has tried to quit many times. Even reducing his nicotine "dosage" significantly affects his mood, sleep, and ability to concentrate at work. He also drinks a good deal of coffee and caffeinated soft drinks. Nicotine and caffeine can be added to the list of drugs he depends on. His psychiatrists have repeatedly urged him to limit his caffeine intake and to exercise regularly. “I’ve done neither,” he told me, with no hint of regret. Adam, it seems, has set rather strict limits on what he is willing to do for his own well-being.

When Adam called after cutting his hand, he asked himself and me why he had acted so “pathetically.” My verbal groping to understand what had happened included the words “the illness.” With more conviction than I have ever heard come from this highly tentative person, Adam shot back, “It’s not the illness, it’s me. That’s the way I’ve been doing things for 16 years.”

Adam was back at work the day after he cut his hand. He felt shaky, but toughed it out, and then took a few days off. He called me the following week. “I’ve been going about this all wrong,” he said. “I have to work on my issues of needing to get attention. When I was a kid my parents felt it was better if I wasn’t heard … In preschool, when the teacher hit me on the head with a ruler, I’d go to the nurse’s office. It was for attention. That’s what happened at the store when I cut my hand.”

But Adam’s insight is transient and limited. Seemingly ignoring the implications of his acknowledged contributions to his illness, he insists he does not see how, if he is taking medication for a possible brain disorder, that illness could be psychological as well. Perhaps Adam resists facing the dynamic component of his illness because he fears what that would require of him. Are there issues he does not want to deal with, emotional scabs he does not want to pick? He often throws out hints about the pain he experienced growing up as he became entangled in family dynamics. His father drank heavily then, and continues to abuse alcohol now, which worries Adam. His mother, he says, overreacts to everything.

Even before the symptoms of his illness appeared, Adam was not comfortable in his own skin. He never felt like he was one of the crowd, though he pretended to be and was always accepted by his peers. He acknowledged hiding behind the image of the prep-school lacrosse player he was. How many other “masks” did Adam wear before that particular one cracked under the pressure of a team practice? Who was he, really, while he was playing competitive sports, serving as president of the student council, and singing for eight years in his church choir?

In my first book, *The Marginal Self*, I drew from the philosophical and literary tradition of existentialism to explore the concepts of selfhood and authenticity. I looked into how a person can live inauthentically, outside his “real self,” through a persona (“mask”) that meets the world, but does not engage real feelings. I coined the term “schizoid erosion of self”[1] to describe how a psyche could be damaged by living in this way. It was easy to find examples of this type of self-destruction in psychological and psychoanalytic writing, as well as in literature and film.

Could Adam's initial paranoid episode and subsequent 16-year psychiatric morbidity be understood as a failure to develop an adequate self and an adult personality? Are his signature paranoia and addictions defenses against the anxiety that is inevitable when an underdeveloped self is stripped of the "mask" that once successfully fronted for it? Perhaps this paranoia is an instance of what Jean-Paul Sartre had in mind when he wrote, "I regard mental illness as the 'way out' that the free organism, in its total unity, invents in order to be able to live through an intolerable situation."[2] It may also be the kind of deviant experience that Alfred Adler was thinking of when he wagered, "Neurosis and psychosis are modes of expression for human beings who have lost courage."[3]

Once, while Adam was talking about how his paranoia could be related to his unwillingness to cope with everyday events, he conceded, "I'm so manipulative." His tone implied that he saw this manipulation as a significant component of his illness. Predictably, each of Adam's paranoid episodes initiates a rescue. Family members, friends, employers, and various clinicians appear and minister to him, relieving him of the obligation of having to cope with whatever it is he finds intolerable at the moment. Some time after he cut his finger at the store, Adam made this related disclosure, which seemed to come from a part of his Being that he was not used to accessing, much less disclosing: "Instead of taking all that medication, I wish I had just dealt with what was going on." I see this cryptic statement as a revelation of Adam's "real self."

Why does Adam reveal himself to me in this way? Clearly, he has the need to tell someone about certain thoughts and feelings that haunt him. He calls me when things get rough, and when he is anxious, depressed, and paranoid (and, I eventually realized, after he uses illicit drugs and feels guilty about it). I am his sounding board, his reality check. He is respectful of my time, and we rarely talk longer than five or ten minutes. I conclude many of the calls by saying, "This is what you should be talking to your psychiatrist and drug counselor about." He agrees, and calls again several days later, with the same questions and the same need for reassurance. Adam is largely opaque to himself.

Besides the fact that little of what I say sticks with him, a likely reason Adam calls me is that he feels he is not getting something he needs from his psychiatrist and his drug counselor. (I am aware of the ego and rescuer factors here, and try to resist these snares.) His psychiatrist sees him every two or three months, and, Adam says, deals mostly with his medication. His drug counselor talks to him about drugs, but nothing else. One can wonder if Adam's clinicians, believing he has a schizophrenia spectrum disorder, have decided that there is no point in exploring this kind of dynamic material with him.[4]

Over a period of several years, my frustration has grown along with Adam's frustration. He isn't getting worse, but he isn't getting better, either. He takes his medication and has not been hospitalized in ten years. But Adam feels he is going nowhere, as he struggles with anxiety, depression, and paranoia. His work at the grocery store is appreciated by his employer and his customers, but the job offers no chance for advancement. Adam has looked for other jobs, and gone on interviews, but quickly recognized that he did not have the education and the emotional capacity for the more challenging work he would like to do. His frustration comes from wanting more from life but knowing that he lacks the resources to get more. In spite of his competence and popularity at the store, his low tolerance for stress and his paranoia often make it hard for him to get through the day. A harsh remark from a coworker can send him home for several days. Fortunately, Adam's employer understands his special circumstances.

I often ruminate over what may have caused Adam's illness. Are his paranoia and the dysfunction that derive from it attributable to the developmentally programmed synaptic misconnections and faulty neurotransmission currently believed to underlie schizophrenia? Or did Adam's long and heavy use of drugs and alcohol damage neurons in his brain and compromise functions that make it possible for a person to be part of a consensually validated reality? This kind of complication occurs with a small percentage of heavy drug users. Certain individuals may be more susceptible to drug-induced neurological trauma than others, and some drugs, or combinations of drugs, are unusually potent neurotoxins. Contaminants can be generated when a drug is made with poor quality control. And sometimes, toxic materials are used to "cut" a drug on the street. Adam admits to using every drug he could find. That degree of usage creates many possibilities for neurotoxicity.

When Adam's anxiety and paranoia reach their zenith, I ask myself if anything short of a psychosis-inducing defect in brain circuitry could explain his thinking, feeling, and behavior. On his better days, I remember that I have seen anxiety alone cripple people in equally bizarre ways. Ultimately, Adam's anxiety lies in not knowing who he is, or being able to find his place in the world. He has made it clear to me that his self-esteem is so low he feels others see him as worthless. It may seem perfectly reasonable to Adam that those who know him in this way would want to annihilate his "worthless" existence. Perhaps his paranoia is a defense that makes others out to be the threat, so he can displace the carnage inside his own psyche.

One would like to know how Adam came to feel this way about himself. Perhaps, during his many years of chemical intoxication, he simply did not do the work of living required to hit the developmental milestones of adolescence and young adulthood that create the psychological structures necessary for an adequate adult personality. This includes what Erik Erikson called the capacity for basic trust, the absence of which is the ground for paranoia.[5] Adam may once have established this trust only to see it erode when he was later distracted from formative life tasks by drugs and alcohol.

Sometimes when Adam calls, he tells me he feels like he is losing his mind. (I have never seen him anywhere near a major decompensation.) After I finish talking him down and return to my own world, I look to the clinicians, philosophers, and neuroscientists who helped shape my thinking about mental illness: Eugen Bleuler spoke of the broken mind of the schizophrenic, Gregory Bateson of a double bind that can cause psychic shearing and may contribute to psychosis,[6] R.D. Laing of the divided self rooted in self-deception,[7] Alfred Adler of lost courage that leads to neurosis and psychosis, Jean-Paul Sartre of the intolerable situation that mental illness allows someone to skirt, Erik Erikson of the basic trust necessary for further stages of development, and the neuroscientists of overactive brain dopamine circuits. I can only wonder where Adam might be in all this.

Three years later...

On a Sunday evening in October 2001, Adam called sounding upbeat but in full control. He retold the story of the episode with his lacrosse coach in 1986, which led to his leaving college during freshman year and to his first hospitalization. And then he revealed a thought he had just after he was admitted to the hospital: "If everybody thinks I'm crazy, I've got a free ride from my parents and the world."

This was something new. Adam was acknowledging that, in spite of the emotional trauma involved in his leaving school and being hospitalized, as well as the impact on his brain of the drugs and alcohol he had been abusing steadily for several years, he was thinking lucidly enough to understand the secondary gain that came with being diagnosed with a mental illness. The expectations of his parents and the rest of the world were now on hold. Adam had reinvented himself as a mental patient. Monkey off his back!

The revelations from that Sunday evening call kept on coming. "I've hit bottom … I need a lot of help … I'm a total addict success … I wanted an easy way out … I believed my own lie." Adam had just returned from a meeting of Narcotics Anonymous and was talking the language of addiction and recovery. Then he addressed these words directly to me: "You're seeing a miracle here. You're seeing a drug addict and alcoholic recover."

I had the distinct impression Adam was telling me he knows something important about himself that I did not know—what made his illness *necessary.* I had long suspected that Adam may have a significant secret he is trying to cover up with his addiction and paranoia. Is that what he meant when he told me earlier, "Instead of taking all that medication, I should have dealt with what was going on"? What is the thing that must not be known?[8] Does Adam harbor rage for his parents because they somehow discouraged him from becoming his own person? Is that how he came to feel like he is nothing? Could he have the kind of sexual feelings he dare not act on because he fears how his parents and friends might react?

And then Adam really got down to it. "I believed my lie so much I lived my lie," he told me. Adam the drug addict was now talking the language of the authentic self. "I watched the other patients in the hospital. I knew how to act and what to say to get Thorazine, Xanax … it was all legit." Adam the drug addict had figured out how to make the doctors give him prescription drugs. Now, with their help, he was a different kind of drug addict.

I believe Adam confided in me, and not in his doctors, because he knew I would not take away his psychiatric diagnoses or his medication. Adam gratefully accepted the identity of a mental patient proffered to him by his psychiatrists: "When they told me I was schizophrenic, I was glad; that was better than being nothing." The door to this particular way of avoiding his authentic self may have been opened many years earlier when an uncle told him, "If you think you are sick, you are sick." Adam acknowledged he had used that excuse to get out of school. And ultimately, it seems, out of his life as well.

At this point I could no longer doubt that, since 1986, Adam had been hiding behind an illness he never had. Meanwhile, the illness he does have—an overarching fear of engaging in the world as he has come to know it—goes unrecognized and untreated. Such was the Faustian deal Adam struck with his psychiatrists. He played his get-out-of-life card and the psychiatrists played their own game back at him. They assumed he had some kind of brain chemical imbalance and medicated him relentlessly, as if some drug or combination of drugs would redress this imbalance and make him well. Instead of taking a stand against what, as Adam put it, "was really going on"—a requirement of effective psychotherapy—his psychiatrists fused with that pathology, in essence aiding and abetting his willful denial of his authentic self.[9]

Adam has what he calls "moments of clarity," when he has some sense of himself as a real person who is capable of making choices. Most of the time, he told me, he feels like an "empty shell." "I know and I don't know" is how he acknowledges the fleeting insight he has into what he has done with his life. I believe that when Adam talks to me in his "I know" mode he is experimenting with an authentic way of being himself, knowing full well that when he hangs up the phone he can return to the self-deceiving safety of "I don't know." I can sense his exhilaration as he briefly experiments with his unmasked self before again retreating behind the mask. I try to encourage Adam's authentic mode, but I am limited in what I can do because I am his friend, not his therapist. According to Adam, in spite of having continuous psychiatric care since 1986, none of his numerous clinicians ever challenged him in this way. "I had good doctors, but they did not help me" was his assessment of the situation. (My impression: Adam played his drug addict cards better than these clinicians played their psychiatrist cards.)

Eventually, Adam told me more about his early life. His father and mother both drank heavily when he was a child. They were socially active and entertained friends and business associates at their large house in an upper-middle-class neighborhood. At age eight, Adam would sneak downstairs after parties his parents had given and drink the wine and hard liquor left in the glasses of the departed guests. Because his parents and their friends seemed to enjoy drinking, Adam got the idea that drinking was a good thing. He told me about an incident that he called a "turning point in my addiction." One evening during the summer of his junior or senior year in high school, Adam was out drinking at a bar with a classmate and came home to get some money. He found his father passed out in the bathroom and his mother drunk upstairs. "Your father will be all right," his mother assured him. "He just had too much to drink." Adam turned to his friend and said "Let's get drunk," which they did.

Adam spoke as if he had learned from his parents that it is acceptable to be drunk. Both of Adam's parents took Valium, though neither was addicted. Adam first dipped into his parents' supply of this tranquilizer at the age of ten. He said he came to believe that using Valium was a valid way to deal with what he was feeling.

Adam has made periodic efforts to taper and stop the medication he has taken continuously since he was first hospitalized. (Most recently, he has been on Prolixin, Wellbutrin, Prozac, and Tegretol.) Twice, he told me, his psychiatrist reduced his Prolixin. But, he explained, "I got nervous and put myself back on the full dosage. That was the drug addict in me." Adam insisted that he did not develop psychotic symptoms while the drug was being tapered. He simply lost his nerve. I believe he has come to feel that he needs psychotropic drugs to regulate his life, just as he concluded earlier that he needed alcohol and Valium. Adam once stopped all his medications on his own, but his mother found out, contacted the psychiatrist and, at a family meeting with the psychiatrist, it was decided that the medication should be resumed. Adam complied.

Adam is afraid of his parents and his psychiatrist, and ultimately bows to their will. "If I fired my psychiatrist, couldn't he have me committed?" he asked, clearly convinced that this could happen. Adam's parents have fears of their own. They are petrified that if Adam reduces or discontinues his medication, he would go back to using drugs and alcohol, lose control of his life, and end up in the hospital again. (Of course, as long as a chemical imbalance is blamed for their son's problematic life, his parents can stay off the hook for what their shortcomings may have contributed to his illness.) One can only wonder what Adam's psychiatrist fears. After being on just about every psychotropic drug in the formulary since 1986, who could predict what rebound symptoms he would experience if he reduced or stopped his current medications? Drugs often mask the rebound symptoms that will appear after that drug is withdrawn.

That Adam should continue to writhe in the chemical and psychological restraint of his medication became even more poignant when, in 2002, the paranoia that had eaten into his life for so long inexplicably disappeared! Ironically, Adam then faced a real challenge at work. A female employee in the store accused him of sexual harassment, a charge that was immediately seen as bogus by the store manager and owner. The obviously disturbed young woman had made similar unsubstantiated charges while working elsewhere. Adam saw the situation for what it was, and reality-tested it as any mentally stable person would have done. Neither his life nor his work suffered because of the accusation. The woman was eventually fired, and Adam was transferred to another branch of the store without penalty or prejudice.

Adam told me—and I believed him—that he has not had any significant paranoid thoughts since 2002. The paranoia did not return even when he was fired from his job in 2003, after he had used cocaine for several weeks and either did not come to work or was compromised by the drug when he did.

When I asked Adam what happened to the paranoia that had colored so much of his adult life he replied, as if he had already given this question some thought, "Maybe I don't need it anymore." Then he quickly added, as if to take back some of his answer, that this might be "too convenient" an explanation. At another time when I asked the same question, he said, "I have too many other things to worry about to be paranoid." Now that Adam's paranoia is history, I am more convinced than ever that it was driven by anxiety, and was psychogenic. My best guess is that, by 2002, Adam had outgrown this defense, which he had clung to for 16 years.

To a clinician following the criteria of the *DSM*-IV—or the *DSM-III* that was being used in 1986 when Adam was diagnosed with schizophrenia—a disturbance at the level of a personality disorder, complicated by severe substance abuse, would seem to adequately account for the clinical facts of Adam's case. (Occam's razor, also known as the principle of parsimony, is satisfied here: when a phenomenon can be explained in several ways, the simplest explanation is most likely to be correct.) The *DSM-IV* defines a personality disorder as "an enduring pattern of inner experience and behavior that deviates markedly from the expectations of the individual's culture, is pervasive and inflexible, has an onset in adolescence or early adulthood, is stable over time, and leads to distress or impairment."[10]

Adam's illness has many features consistent with avoidant, dependent, histrionic, borderline, and paranoid personality disorders. Personality disorder traits are know to lessen, or "burn out," over time, and that may be what happened with Adam's paranoia. The *DSM-II* (but not the *DSM-IV*) includes the diagnosis of inadequate personality disorder, which seems to describe Adam quite accurately: "This behavior pattern is characterized by ineffectual responses to emotional, social, intellectual and physical demands. While the patient seems neither physically or mentally deficient, he does manifest inadaptability, ineptness, poor judgment, social instability, and lack of physical and emotional stamina."[11] Adam could have been made from this formula. What a pity the inadequate personality is no longer recognized by the official lexicon of psychopathology. How many other "inadequate" patients have been punished with a diagnosis of a more severe mental illness they did not have and been medicated for it?

In retrospect, the diagnoses of schizophrenia, then bipolar disorder and, finally, schizoaffective disorder that Adam was given seem to have come from an almost willful disregard by his psychiatrists of the facts of his case. Instead of listening with the clinician's "third ear"[12] for the subtext of Adam's story, these psychiatrists effectively closed their ears and insisted that he had a brain illness that could be alleviated only with multiple psychotropic drugs. Of course, in conceiving of Adam's illness as they did, the psychiatrists unwittingly gave him another card to play in the elaboration of that illness—the mental health card! Even after Adam had stopped being paranoid—and held that advance for two years—his psychiatrist stood behind his diagnosis of schizoaffective disorder and refused to support Adam's wish to taper his medication.

CHAPTER 6
How Psychiatry Created an Epidemic of Misdiagnosed Bipolar Disorder

After working in the emergency room for several years, I began to suspect that most of the patients I was seeing there who had been previously diagnosed with bipolar disorder did not have this mental illness. The feel and gestalt of their stories led me to believe that their psychological and physiological "lesions" did not go that deep. When I asked my reputed bipolar patients if they had ever felt, thought, or behaved in ways that would satisfy the *DSM-IV* criteria for hypomania or mania, perhaps one in five responded affirmatively. The others often sent back looks of disbelief. When I asked if they thought they had bipolar disorder, I got this spectrum of answers: Yes ... That's what the doctor said ... I don't know ... You're the doctor, you tell me ... No. Most of these patients had little insight into what their real problems were or what they could be doing to help themselves. That they had been misdiagnosed did not seem to concern them at all.

Alicia, a 19-year-old college sophomore, was brought to the ER by her mother after being contacted by Alicia's roommates. Earlier, at a party, Alicia was rudely spoken to and then pushed by a football player whom she knew. She became angry and had a verbal outburst. Back at her apartment, she made several superficial cuts to her left ventral wrist.

Often before I interview a patient, a member of the ER staff will tell me that someone who has just been seen has a "flat affect." Usually, patients who start out with a leaden face brighten up once the interview starts. But Alicia, who had looked "flat" to the nurse, stayed flat—facially, vocally, and in every other way her body could signal that she was severely depressed.

She rarely looked directly at me, though I repeatedly urged her to do so, explaining how I find it hard to talk to patients when they turn away.

Alicia told me that she had been depressed for most of her life. During the last five years, she had periodically made cuts to her arms and legs. When I tried to get a sense of how constant and pervasive her depression was, she told me that she usually feels bad, and feels good only for short periods, and then only after she accomplishes something significant. Then her mood reverts back to dysthymia or depression. Alicia reported chronic poor sleep, which had become worse recently, and reduced appetite. She had never felt worse than on the day I talked to her.[1] Alicia denied that the cuts she had been making to her arms and legs during the last five years were intended to end her life or that she ever wanted, or tried, to kill herself. She had never had any experiences that could be considered psychotic.

Alicia's blood alcohol level (BAL) was 121 mg/dL. She acknowledged occasionally drinking to the point of intoxication, as well as using marijuana sporadically since high school. Her toxicology screen was negative for marijuana and other drugs of abuse. She had no significant medical problems.

Alicia was an only child and was raised in a middle-class household. Some time between the age of 3 and 5, she was forced into a sexual act by the grandson of a babysitter, who was about 12 years old at the time. Alicia made it clear that she did not want to talk about what had happened.

Alicia was passive and had to be repeatedly prodded to engage in the interview. She did not seem interested in talking about the events that changed the course of her evening, or appear to be at all concerned that she was in the ER. In fact, she gave the impression that all this was happening to someone else, not to her. She seemed fully resigned to her saturnine fate.[2] When I asked if the detachment she was showing during the interview was usual for her, she responded, "Most of my life I have hidden behind a façade." She explained that she often wore a happy face to hide her pain and emptiness. This acknowledgment was my entry point into Alicia's life.

Alicia hoped to study journalism, but she had never been a good student and withdrew from all her classes two months earlier. Increasing anger and depression made it impossible for her to do the required work. She lived in an apartment off campus with three other female students whom she had known for several years. She had not yet had a serious boyfriend. Easily and with no evident sign of regret, she told me, "I'm a virgin."

Whatever my doubts may have been about Alicia's having what the *DSM-IV* calls borderline personality disorder disappeared after I spoke to her mother in the waiting room. Alicia had vigorously denied to me that she missed having her father in her life or that his absence had anything to do with her being angry and depressed. The mother lost no time in correcting this misstatement, insisting that what Alicia saw as the father's abandonment was a constant source of anguish to her daughter. Alicia's chronic depression was starting to sound like the "abandonment depression"[3] that many borderline patients experience.

Another significant point of contention for Alicia was her mother's supposed failure to recognize, and presumably to do anything about, Alicia's life-long cover-up of her real feelings. The mother said her daughter had angrily thrown this issue back at her many times. Clearly, Alicia had been playing a big-time blame game with both of her parents. Anger and retribution are key borderline traits and have been labeled by the psychoanalyst James F. Masterson as the "talionic impulse."[4]

When I asked Alicia's mother why she thought her daughter was having trouble now, she responded: "Alicia has problems being an adult. She can't handle the academic pressure of school or the social pressure, either." Alicia had taken driving lessons, but did not get her license. "She's afraid to drive a car," the mother told me. The adult world, with its expectations and responsibilities, was impinging hard on Alicia and asking her to do things she could not see her way to doing. Alicia was paying a higher price now—most noticeably in increased anger, depression, and emotional numbness and isolation—for the inauthentic life of avoidance she had lived all along. She had little insight into how all this had happened to her and no plan to fix any of it.

Two weeks earlier, Alicia had been diagnosed with bipolar disorder by a psychiatrist, and prescribed Depakote. How a 19-year-old female with mood swings that did not include any of the features of hypomania or mania; who was sexually abused at a young age; who felt abandoned by her father and betrayed by her mother; who lived with chronic feelings of detachment and emptiness; who experienced worsening anger and depression; who avoided a serious relationship with a significant other; who showed a general unwillingness to take on the responsibilities of adult life; and who reported a five-year history of self-mutilation could be diagnosed with and medicated for bipolar disorder is difficult to understand. During our interview, Alicia gave a virtual poster presentation on borderline pathology.[5]

Whenever I interview an ER patient who reports a prior bipolar diagnosis—and that's about one half of the patients I see—I ask the questions from the *DSM-IV* that would either establish or rule out hypomania or mania.[6] As I put each of these questions to Alicia, she responded wholeheartedly in the negative (interesting, because her answers to most of the other questions were decidedly half-hearted). She vigorously denied ever having been in a heightened, expansive, or euphoric mood. Her mood ranged from normal good (when she felt she was accomplishing something special, which, no doubt, distracted her from her base-line feeling of emptiness) to dysthymia (which is how she felt most of the time) to varying degrees of depression (which is how she had been feeling for the last few months). Later, when I interviewed the mother, I went through the same list of questions, and got the same negative replies. "That's not my daughter," Alicia's mother insisted.

Alicia met none of the criteria for bipolar disorder and all of the borderline personality disorder criteria. I now had a choice to make. I could keep quiet and refer the patient back to a psychiatrist whom I knew had made a mistake that would undermine Alicia's treatment. But who would I be serving by doing this? Certainly not the patient, whose well-being I was supposed to be advocating for. I rejected silence and informed Alicia and her mother that I felt the bipolar diagnosis was wrong. When I gave her the news, Alicia, who had just been evaluated by her third psychiatrist, replied, "I've been told different things by different doctors. Some say unipolar depression, some say bipolar." Alicia was nonplussed, and didn't appear to care what kind of mental disorder she had. The mother's response was more committal: "But [the psychiatrist] has such good credentials," she wanted me to know, dropping the name of a medical school that is indeed highly regarded. "The doctor said she was convinced that Alicia was bipolar and that giving her an antidepressant might make her psychotic."

Having questioned my own motivation in deciding to reveal what I considered a misdiagnosis, I now wondered what had motivated Alicia's psychiatrist. Was this clinician with the "good credentials" subconsciously playing it safe? Was she blinded to a diagnosis that should have been obvious by the fear that Alicia's emotional brittleness might derive from a bipolar diathesis, driven by a chemical imbalance whose manifestations could be made more severe with an antidepressant? (Many patients with bipolar disorder can take antidepressants safely and with good results, but some do become manic and psychotic.) Had Alicia's psychiatrist seen her patient's anger and irritability, even in the absence of elevated mood, as pathognomonic for bipolar disorder, rather than as the sentinel symptoms of borderline personality disorder as I had? This would explain her prescribing a usually well-tolerated mood stabilizer, rather than an often more problematic antidepressant.

My guess is that Alicia's anger and depression were rooted in her failure to successfully negotiate the challenges and conflicts she met as she made her way through childhood and adolescence. Instead, she appeared to have lived out a good deal of this experience in a pathological way, failing to overcome what she felt was bad about the hand life had dealt her—the sexual abuse, her father's abandonment, and her mother's failure to affirm her real self. Alicia had numbed herself to the inauthentic life she was living, cutting her arms and legs so she could feel *something* as she looked to the bleeding cuts, and the pain they caused, for proof that she existed.[7]

Considering Alicia's lifelong and worsening depression, an antidepressant might have been the better choice for a first-line drug. According to her mother, Alicia was calmer since starting Depakote, though apparently not calm enough to keep her from cutting her wrist after being badly treated by a football player at a party. In the ER, Alicia had only 22 mcg/mL of valproic acid, Depakote's active agent, in her blood, a subtherapeutic level (therapeutic range 50–100 mcg/mL). I warned her about the danger of mixing Depakote with the amount of alcohol she used the night I saw her.

Alicia planned to spend the next few days at her mother's house and then return to her apartment and her friends. I recommended that they call her psychiatrist later that day (we finished the evaluation around 6:00 a.m.). Ideally, Alicia should have a clinician who was trained to do intensive psychotherapy, and is dedicated to doing it over the long haul. I also recommended getting another opinion on the diagnosis, and suggested that they call a local psychiatric hospital for a referral. I felt fairly confident that Alicia's mother would make sure her daughter followed through.

Alicia's misdiagnosis was a mistake ready to happen. If patients are angry and irritable, have frequent changes in mood, and spend more money or engage in more sex than their clinicians think is prudent, a bipolar diagnosis is likely. These patients are getting what I have come to see as the "bipolar dispensation." This has something in it for everyone involved. Patients can avoid seeing their problem as originating in a pathological misuse of their freedom, a situation that would require work on their part to change; mom and dad can skip the test of being Winnicott's "good-enough" parents;[8] a culture and society that incline its citizens toward an inauthentic life goes unchallenged; and physicians who prescribe the medication for a purported bipolar illness can do three med checks an hour, earning a respectable reimbursement from managed care, which would not pay them comparably for a 50-minute therapy hour.

Calling Alicia bipolar is meaningless, and a disservice. Blaming her pathological thinking, feeling, and behavior on a chemical imbalance labels her as damaged in a way and to a degree that she is not damaged. At the same time, Alicia is kept from addressing what has really gone wrong in her life.

In psychiatry, as everywhere else, success breeds imitators. Mood-stabilizing drugs, from the original lithium carbonate to an ever-expanding line of anticonvulsants, have made life livable for many with true bipolar disorder. This mental disorder is most likely caused by a brain chemical imbalance that, in effect, autonomously dictates the affected person's mood. A chemical agent is required to rectify the imbalance. The *DSM-IV* designates this illness as bipolar I. To meet criteria, someone must have at least one full manic episode (without the specified exclusion factors) that alternates with episodes of major depression. Ironically, here is an instance where the *DSM* could be genuinely useful, and it is almost universally ignored.[9]

In *An Unquiet Mind*, a beautifully written book that describes her own bipolar I illness, the psychologist Kay Redfield Jamison makes it clear that had it not been for lithium, she would have lost not only her career, but her life as well. Bipolar II disorder, which is rarely ever specified as such in patients' charts and records, is said by the *DSM-IV* to be a parallel cycling of mood where hypomania, a lesser and sometimes adaptive state of chemically driven high mood, takes the place of full-blown mania. Though these two illnesses are spoken of and written about as if they were dimensionally related, there is as yet no empirical evidence that bipolar II is a milder version of bipolar I.[10]

As evidence accumulated that mood-stabilizing drugs calmed patients down, clinicians began to conflate the mood swings of those who had true bipolar I disorder with a different kind of mood swing that is often experienced by those who habitually use immature or primitive defenses and face the world with an alienated, anxious, and brittle self. Many of these patients have Axis II personality disorders—especially the cluster B disorders: antisocial, borderline, histrionic, narcissistic—with psychodynamics that make a pathological variation in mood inevitable. Anger, irritability, and grandiosity are all characteristics of Axis II disorders. Once called neurosis or character disorder, this kind of pathological behavior is now often misread as a manifestation of hypomania or mania.

The essential differential call to be made when patients experience alternating extremes of mood is between bipolar disorder, a primary, Janus-faced chemical imbalance resulting in mania, coupled with major depression, and another kind of cyclic mood disturbance that is driven mainly by pathological psychodynamics.[11]

To be able to make this call, a diagnostician must understand and recognize the psychodynamics of Axis II disorders, and how patients with these disorders construct their lives in ways that are bound to generate fluctuating mood states.[12] One can wonder if Alicia's psychiatrist, who had "good credentials," had spent enough time with the challenging texts that must be mastered before a clinician is able to correctly diagnose and effectively treat Axis II pathology. Some psychiatry residency programs present all mental illness as a primary disturbance of the brain's biological substrate and do not bother with this kind of training, or offer it only as an afterthought. Many clinicians practicing now diagnose solely by matching their patients' symptoms to the *DSM-IV*'s behavioral criteria. Medication is then used to treat these symptoms without the clinician ever understanding the provenance and meaning of the patient's pathological behavior.

For the well-being of patients and for its own integrity as a profession, psychiatry needs to specify more stringently the feeling states and behaviors that may be called bipolar disorder. The designation of bipolar I (with mania) and bipolar II (with hypomania) should be limited to what can be clinically inferred as chemically induced mood disorders (there are no markers, lab tests. or brain scans to help here). Lacking primary psychodynamic roots, these mood states seem to be driven by an autonomous pathophysiological process that overrides the normal dialectic between the choices people make—whatever their level of awareness is about what they are doing—and the way they subsequently feel.

The bipolar I or bipolar II appellations should not be used to name mood swings that are often part and parcel of Axis II, substance abuse, and anxiety disorders. Nor should these diagnoses be given to people with mercurial personalities, who often have rapid changes in mood but are otherwise "normal," or to those whose mood fluctuates more than usual as they come up against unusually difficult situations. Finally, the bipolar diagnosis should be withheld in patients who appear to live out a pervasive, world-transforming anger. Psychiatry has yet to acknowledge and investigate the structure and behavioral manifestations of pathological anger, which generates turbulent swings in mood that are often misread as hypomania or mania.

I suspect that the *DSM-IV*'s Criterion A, which allows "irritable" mood to be substituted for "elevated or expansive" mood, is the rationale (perhaps rationalization would be a better word) for a good deal of bipolar misdiagnosis. Persons with Axis II disorders, and those who abuse drugs and alcohol, are intrinsically irritable, though most never develop hypomania or mania. Above all, we need to get rid of the notion that, ipso facto, mood swings always imply a primary biochemical derangement of the brain. Mood stabilizers, neuroleptics, and atypical antipsychotics can be used to treat symptoms such as anxiety, agitation, and severe insomnia without first misdiagnosing bipolar disorder as a justification.

To grasp what the elevated/expansive/irritable deformation of mood known as mania really is, a clinician needs to see a certain number of classic manic patients, and to follow them through hospitalization as their condition remits.[13] For an experienced clinician, classical mania is often a straightforward clinical call, but psychopathology does not always present classically. There are patients whose mood swings occupy a middle ground between a primary mood disorder and a disorder driven by psychodynamics. Even an acutely manic patient is capable of what

David S. Janowsky calls "interpersonal maneuvers."[14] These acts involve a purposeful exercise of freedom and choice, though this freedom is attenuated by a compromised biological substrate. Self-deception and manipulation are not strangers to the manic state. The larger point here is that bipolar I patients can still make inauthentic choices that contribute to their pathology at the extremes of their mood swings. With these patients, the art of diagnosis will be pushed to, and at times beyond its limits. The hope is that at least the most egregious bipolar misdiagnoses—like Alicia's—can be avoided.

Ross J. Baldessarini, a biological psychiatrist, psychopharmacologist, and professor of psychiatry at Harvard Medical School, has asked psychiatrists to avoid what he calls a "premature and potentially misleading widening and dilution of the bipolar disorder concept."[15] He points out that "it is hardly surprising that affective instability and fluctuations of mood can be found in many, if not most, other disorders."

> Reasons for urging restraint include the strong impression that classic bipolar disorders—an abundance of phenocopies, notwithstanding—are about as close to a "disease" as we have in modern psychiatry. At least, bipolar disorder offers hope of being a coherent and tractable phenotypic target for genetic, biological, and experimental therapeutic studies. It would be tragic to weaken the disorder just as it is gaining the serious clinical and research attention that it has so long deserved.[16]

An example of the kind of symptom inflation I see all the time in the ER is what happens when patients, often brought in by the police on emergency petition, display what seems to be an unbearable dissatisfaction with their lives. Of course, the ER staff has its own way of expressing dissatisfaction with patients who are loud, belligerent, hard to control, and not redirectable. When patients get out of hand, I routinely hear technicians, nurses, social workers, and attendings use words such as "escalating," "crazy," "tangential," "flight of ideas," "insane," "manic," and "psychotic." In fact, these patients are often just pissed off—and usually for reasons that are not hard to understand. They have not been handling their situations well, and that is why they are in the ER. Often, patients who are extremely anxious can look floridly psychotic.

I suspect that many of the bipolar diagnoses struck in consulting rooms, community mental health centers, and psychiatric hospitals originate in a similar kind of overreaction to patients' misunderstood erratic behavior. As happened with Alicia, language slips and slides to the point where the resulting diagnosis—which always depends on the meaning behind the words used in making it—is meaningless. The separation of symptoms from what European phenomenological psychiatrists call "intentionality" has drastically eroded the standard of care in the diagnosis of mental disorders. (Now, the misdiagnosis of bipolar disorder *is* the standard of care.) Intentionality implies that, in being conscious, a person is always conscious *of* something.[17] This amounts to an ontological guarantee that all conscious activity has meaning, and that all human behavior is purposeful.

Psychiatric diagnosis increasingly suffers from what, in a variety of contexts, has been called "definitional creep."[18] This is a situation where a word or term defined in one way overflows the meaning intended, to include new meanings that range far from the original definition. Definitional creep implies distortion, and that is surely what has happened in the diagnosis of bipolar disorder. For decades, the prevalence of bipolar disorder has been cited as about 1%, the same as for schizophrenia. There is no way to know how many patients are misdiagnosed with this illness now.

The following story came to me through a psychiatric nurse who worked on the inpatient unit of a local hospital. A patient hospitalized there with major depression was given an antidepressant and, several days later, reported that he felt "better than he ever felt before." The psychiatrist immediately concluded that this mood elevation indicated hypomania or mania, diagnosed bipolar disorder, and started the patient on Depakote. Never mind that the *DSM-IV* emphatically proscribes making the bipolar diagnosis under these circumstances, even with hypomania or mania, which the nurse assured me were not in the picture.[19] The patient simply felt "better." Partisans of the statistical approach will argue that this observation is a study with only one subject, but the fact that such a call could be made at all by a licensed, board-certified psychiatrist, who had least 25 years of clinical experience under his belt, makes us stop and ask, What air is psychiatry breathing these days?

Bipolar disorder should be a diagnosis of exclusion, and made only after other, lesser, diagnoses fail to account for a patient's thinking, feeling, and behavior. As specific as the *DSM-IV* is about ruling out other explanations for mood swings, this caveat is widely ignored. As clinicians, it is our job to challenge patients' pathology and to show them how to take a stand against what is wrong in their lives, and not to encourage them to believe they have a more serious kind of pathology.

This is precisely what happened to Angela, a woman who was referred to a private practice group I worked for several years ago. Angela's insurance carrier was changed, and she could no longer see the psychiatrist who, ten years earlier, had diagnosed her as manic depressive and prescribed lithium. Married, with an adolescent daughter, Angela was then in her mid-fifties. She had been a nun, but left the order when she was in her late twenties. Her chief complaints at the time she started working with me were serious conflicts with her husband and daughter, as well as feelings of regret that she had not lived her life well.

Everything Angela said and did felt like drama. She came across as all froth and no substance. She was shallow, self-centered, and selfish. Her husband did not make much money, but Angela felt no obligation to contribute to the family finances. She would always find some reason why a job she had was not worthy of her, and quit. She missed no chance to tell me how inadequate her husband was, and that included his inability to satisfy her sexually.

I questioned Angela about her mood. It did not take much prodding to discover that she had never had a manic episode, or even any manic symptoms. Nor had she experienced any mood variations that could be stretched to hypomania. Angela's depressions were in the mild to moderate range of severity and never lasted more than a few days. Her mood swings consisted of these down periods, which reverted to a state of euthymic dissatisfaction and frustration, and then went down again, usually after she became more than usually upset about how her life was going. Angela had never had psychotic symptoms or been hospitalized for a mental disorder. She denied ever using illicit drugs or abusing alcohol.

Angela was not, and had never been, manic depressive. Without doubt, she did make the *DSM-IV* criteria for histrionic personality disorder. She also had some narcissistic features. For ten years, Angela's psychiatrist had told her that her problems came from a chemical imbalance in her brain and that the only thing she could do was take lithium, which she did. During that time, Angela lost any chance she might have had to address the real issues that diminished her life and the lives of her long-suffering husband and daughter, who believed Angela had a brain disorder and that she was not responsible for her destructive behavior.

To make sure that I wasn't missing anything, I called the psychiatrist who had granted Angela's "bipolar dispensation," making possible her gratuitous life as a manic depressive. He told me essentially the same story that Angela had told me. He also stuck to his diagnosis, even after I gave him my reasons for believing that it was incorrect. Then he informed me that he had done a part of his psychiatric training at a famous medical institution and was on the committee that set the *DSM-III* criteria for mood disorders! Looking back, I suppose he was telling me that he had "good credentials."

I asked the psychiatrist from our group who was managing Angela's medication for another opinion on her diagnosis. He concurred that Angela had never met the criteria for bipolar disorder. As I supported her in our sessions, the lithium was tapered. Angela tolerated the drug reduction fairly well, though her anxiety increased. She did not become manic, hypomanic, or depressed, but she began to feel guilty about the pain she had caused her family.

About three months after we started working together, Angela went to another hospital for an outpatient gynecological procedure. She must have put on quite a display of histrionics there because at our next meeting she told me that her gynecologist had said, "I'm not letting you out of here until you see a psychiatrist." An appointment was made, and Angela kept it. A few days later, she called to thank me for all I had done for her and informed me that she was continuing her psychiatric treatment at the other hospital.

No one—not the mental health care profession, not the law, not even the patient—has much interest in holding a clinician responsible for making a wrong bipolar diagnosis. No one says: this is wrong … you missed the patient here … this diagnosis makes it impossible for the patient to see and confront what is really going on … you did not play by the rules as we know them. There is a certain cachet to being bipolar now, as if this were an honorable way of being mentally ill. The diagnosis often serves as an explanation, as well as a justification, for a person's unacceptable behavior. When one of my ER patients was told that he was bipolar (incorrectly, I believe), his psychiatrist tried to reassure him by disclosing that he, too, was bipolar.

Clinicians are reluctant to change a patient's bipolar disorder or schizophrenia diagnosis. I have seen patients who were wrongly diagnosed 5, 10, 15, and 20 years earlier live with these labels, often not understanding what they meant. Some took the medication prescribed, others did not. All were poorly served by a profession that is supposed to help patients get it right after they themselves got it wrong the first time.

Sadly—ironically—some patients whose lives are amorphous and chaotic use their wrong diagnosis as a way to seed the only identity they will ever know. A mental disorder misdiagnosed in a vulnerable patient can induce the patient to create the symptoms of that disorder. This is a particular example of a general phenomenon that the philosopher Ian Hacking called "dynamic nominalism."[20] Hacking saw that by giving people a name they can identify with, some will choose to live that way.

CHAPTER 7

Willing Psychotic Symptoms

Psychotic symptoms—delusions, hallucinations, paranoia, thought disorder—are mostly attributed now to aberrations in brain structure and function. The iconic "chemical imbalance," thought to be a consequence of wrongly wired neural circuits and faulty receptor activity, is seen as an essential component in the distortions of thinking, feeling, and behavior that are different enough from the norm to merit the designation *psychotic*.

The physiological derangement that sometimes occurs in those who use drugs such as amphetamine, lysergic acid diethylamide (LSD), and phencyclidine (PCP) is a known cause of psychosis. So, too, are certain derangements of electrolyte, endocrine, and metabolic functions. Biological psychiatry, the dominant paradigm in mental health now, has extrapolated this association between a known, and sometimes measurable, chemical imbalance and psychosis to explain delusions and hallucinations of unknown pathogenesis that are part and parcel of some mental disorders.[1] In this model, the mind becomes a somewhat passive theater of the brain's "chemical imbalance," ineluctably producing pathological thought, emotion, and behavior.

Not so fast. This story about an elderly woman, whose behavior would be considered paranoid and delusional by any standard, challenges us to reconsider the need to invoke a chemical imbalance to explain all psychotic symptoms.[2]

"Mrs. K," who is 95, lives alone in a ranch-style house on half an acre of land in a rural suburb. On most days during the spring, summer, and fall when the weather is good, Mrs. K works outdoors in the garden. During the winter, when the snow is six inches or less, Mrs. K shovels the driveway out to the road; after heavier accumulations she calls in someone with a plow. This 95-year-old woman never complains about having to cope with the long, cold winters.

Mrs. K pays her own bills and never overdraws her checking account. She prefers to spend most of her time alone and encourages only occasional, short visits from family members. She has no friends and wants none, even though neighbors occasionally make overtures to her. She keeps up with the outside world by watching the news on cable TV. In 1986, Mrs. K's husband died suddenly from heart failure. She has never shown any sign of mourning and, in fact, seemed rejuvenated by her husband's death. Though Mrs. K values life in her advancing years and takes good care of herself, she has made it clear that she is not afraid to die.

Mrs. K has a good quality of life and can still do many of the things that were always important to her. Her sense of the world is largely intact. She appears thin and frail, but for a nonagenarian her health is good. Her close vision has deteriorated and she can no longer sew, but beyond six feet she sees well. She takes 81 mg of aspirin every other day, and receives monthly subcutaneous injections of vitamin B_{12} and folic acid. Mrs. K has had occasional chest pains since her mid-eighties, which her doctor attributes to angina. Sometime after that she was found to have atrial fibrillation. Her only prescription medications are Cardizem and Plavix.

Mrs. K has a son and a daughter, both in their sixties. The daughter and her four grown children live nearby; the son lives in a distant city. The daughter, who is divorced, does Mrs. K's grocery shopping and drives her to doctors' appointments.

Cognitively, Mrs. K is intact—except for this one glitch: She claims to believe that her grandchildren come in the middle of the night, or when she is away during the day, to steal her possessions and that her daughter knows and approves of this. The "stolen" items include sheets, towels, pots and pans, milk, and orange juice. According to Mrs. K, her sterling silver and antiques are being sold and replaced with cheaper items by her grandchildren so they can pocket the difference. These accusations have been made time and again, over a period of many years. Mrs. K also claims that her phone is being tapped. She puts all the blame for this intrusion on her grandchildren and does not feel that either the phone company or the government is involved. According to Mrs. K, the grandchildren listen in on her phone calls because they want to know when she is going to sell her house and when they will get their inheritance.

Mrs. K alleges that her grandchildren steal from her and covet her money because things are not going well for them. Being reminded that three of the grandchildren have good jobs and that the fourth has a husband who makes a respectable living does not sway Mrs. K from this belief. She has been able to convince herself that her grandchildren need the money they steal from her to survive, and that she is their savior. Mrs. K's apparent hatred for her family, manifested in many ways over many years, appears to be transformed through this self-deception into an act of *their* betrayal. The ultimate reason for this woman's hatred is opaque, but there has always been something about her family being successful and happy that has threatened her and tweaked her envy.

The roots to Mrs. K's ambivalence about her family go back decades. After bestowing some favor on her son or daughter she would frequently ask, "Why am I doing this for you?" as if the answer were not apparent to her. She seemed to give with one hand only to take back with the other. On her daughter's wedding day, as the bride walked from the church toward the limousine that was taking the couple to the reception, Mrs. K was heard to say, "I'm sorry I ever let that girl get married." The ceremony had gone well and no one could have known at the time that the groom, a lawyer who was on his way to a successful career, was also on his way to a confrontation with alcohol that would eventually end his career, as well as his marriage. When Mrs. K's son was in grammar school she told him, "Nothing you do will ever make any difference to me." On several occasions at that time she also said, "One day you will come home and find me dead on the floor, with the gas on." By any standard, this is nasty, cruel stuff.

Mrs. K clearly meets criteria for what the *DSM-IV* designates as delusional disorder, persecutory type.[3] Though she has often directed outbursts of anger tinged with paranoia at family members, she has never shown any indication of being clinically depressed, or even of having had a sustained period of low mood. No case can be made for psychotic depression. Mrs. K has never been manic or hypomanic. Neither she nor any of her blood relatives have ever been diagnosed with or treated for a mental disorder.

In *Paradise Lost*, the English poet John Milton (1608–1674) explicitly acknowledged the mind's role in the creation of human experience: "The mind is its own place, and to itself / Can make a heav'n of hell, or a hell of heav'n."[4] Closer to our own time, existential philosophers have argued that, by and large, we are free to create and re-create ourselves and to construct our own world, and, in the process create our own heaven or hell, as circumstances allow. Clinicians who subscribe to this idea see many mental disorders as deriving from self-deceiving, inauthentic modes of what the philosopher Martin Heidegger called our Being-in-the-World (the hyphens here are meant to emphasize the dialectical interaction and inseparability of person and world).[5]

It seems reasonable to ask whether a willed distortion and deformation of a person's "worlded" Being could itself be so significant as to produce psychotic thinking, feeling, and behavior.[6] A psychosis originating in this way would be a dimensional phenomenon, having meaning and structure, and would be a primary function of the mind, though one that, like all mental activity, also has a brain neural substrate. Those who create a paranoid psychosis as their (indirectly, subconsciously) chosen mode of Being-in-the-World can be seen as making the kind of uncalled for connections, as well as the inevitable enemies, that those who live in the consensually validated world choose not to make.

The Jungian analyst John Perry understands paranoia as a weakening of the ego's rational controls, where the id breaks through to take charge: "Energy goes out of the ego into the subconscious, which then becomes the person's whole world."[7] Mrs. K's accusations have a nightmarish, diabolical quality. This part of her world is not controlled by reason, but by primitive processes set loose by what appears to be hatred of her family. Their attempts to demonstrate the absurdity of her taunts are immediately and vigorously absorbed into her existing delusional belief, and neutralized by it. Carl Jung felt that people with delusions are "consumed by a desire to create a new world system … that will enable them to assimilate unknown psychic phenomena and so adapt themselves to their own world."[8] Mrs. K may wish to perceive and relate to her family on her own, delusional terms so as to exert a degree of control over them that she would not otherwise have. Her delusion isolates her from her family, but that may also suit her purpose. It seems that Mrs. K is crazy like a fox. She is as crazy as she *needs* to be, but no crazier.

I have worked with patients whose paranoia, I was certain, was due to anxiety. Mrs. K's paranoia has always seemed to peak at times when things were going well for her family, as if what was good for them was bad for her. The Cardizem that she takes was started by her doctor after a festive get-together of family and friends at her home culminated in an ER visit: chest pain, shortness or breath, lightheadedness, and tachycardia came on suddenly at the height of the celebration. Her indisposition was most likely her body responding to the anxiety of a perceived threat from her happy family with the somatic symptoms of a panic attack (her first). After that, Mrs. K had no more family get-togethers and no more panic attacks.

Paranoid delusions have been challenged with psychotherapy. R.D. Laing saw schizophrenic patients as "divided selves" who had cracked psychically under the stress of family and social pressures.[9] (The literal meaning of the Greek-derived *schizophrenia* is "divided mind.") Taking a page from the existential philosopher Jean-Paul Sartre, Laing understood psychosis as "*a special strategy that a person invents in order to live in an unlivable situation*" (original italics).[10] Laing put as much blame for this break from reality—in what, paradoxically, he saw more as a breakthrough than a breakdown—on pressures external to the patient as on the patient's inability to deal authentically with these pressures and overcome them. At his Tavistock Clinic in London he explored therapeutic techniques to heal what was "divided" in patients who had delusions and hallucinations.

Though several models for treating patients with persecutory delusions have been proposed, there are no published reports to substantiate the effectiveness of these methods.[11] If Mrs. K were to be seen now by a psychiatrist, she would in all likelihood be told that she has a "chemical imbalance" and be encouraged to take antipsychotic medication—in spite of the fact that these drugs have a poor track record in eliminating her type of delusion. To Mrs. K, the thought that anything might be wrong with her is unimaginable, and she would bristle at the suggestion that she is at fault in any way. In fact, the only fault anyone has ever heard Mrs. K acknowledge is that she has done too much for her family. Even if she would agree to seek help for her "problem," it is unlikely that, in the current therapeutic climate, any clinician would dare to challenge this woman's vital lie—the lie she needs to survive. No doubt, Mrs. K will take these paranoid delusions to her grave.

Biological psychiatrists would argue that Mrs. K's paranoia was due to a primary brain disorder, rather than to a functional disorder that is willed and originates in what existential philosophers and clinicians call an *intentional* act that has meaning and purpose. To justify a biological provenance for Mrs. K's behavior, the following question would have to be answered: How does Mrs. K's brain know to select only her family as a target for her paranoia, sparing from accusation almost everyone else in her life? Which neural circuits and neurotransmitters subserve this selection and its behavioral consequences? These questions beg for answers.

John Nash is considered to be one of the great mathematical minds of the twentieth century. A Princeton PhD at age 21, he is best known for developing the mathematics of game theory that was later used to plan military and economic strategy. He won the Nobel Prize for economics in 1994. During the 1950s, while he was still producing what was considered brilliant work, his thinking, feeling, and behavior became unaccountably bizarre, and he was eventually diagnosed with paranoid schizophrenia. Nash angrily resigned his positions at Princeton and the Massachusetts Institute of Technology, making bizarre accusations against his stunned colleagues. His wife was not spared from his paranoid rage, and after standing by him for many years, she divorced him. He floundered badly, could not do any sustained mathematical work, or teach, and lost the ability to function socially.

Nash had paranoid and grandiose delusions and auditory hallucinations. He came to believe that extraterrestrials were sending him messages and that the course of his life was being determined by certain sequences and patterns of numbers. He showed a partial response to Thorazine and Stelazine, but refused to take antipsychotic drugs after 1970. In the mid-1980s, after three decades of a serious mental illness that required many hospitalizations, Nash mysteriously got over the worst of his illness and reclaimed a part of his life and his work.

In 1998, Sylvia Nasar published a widely praised biography of Nash, *A Beautiful Mind*.[12] She carefully parsed every phase of Nash's life, showcasing his brilliance, nobility, and tragedy. It is clear from Nasar's book that, during the prodromal phase of his illness, Nash was anxious and overwhelmed by the pressures of work and marriage, as well as by the conflict he seems to have felt about his homoerotic attachments. He had always been considered aloof and eccentric, and may well have been schizoid or schizotypal before his decompensation. The weight of the evidence in Nasar's book is consistent with the notion that Nash chose to escape his anxiety by creating a world where he was all but omnipotent and everyone was against him. This scenario fits Laing's take on schizophrenia as a strategy invented to live through an intolerable situation.

But let John Nash speak for himself. In the spring of 2002, PBS aired a TV program on Nash titled *A Beautiful Madness*. Nash provided some insightful sound bytes, including this one: "To some extent sanity is a form of conformity. People are always selling the idea that people with mental illness are suffering. I think madness can be an escape. If things are not so good, you maybe want to imagine something better. In madness, I thought I was the most important person in the world."[13] Nash seems to be saying here that he rejected the rational world after it became too painful for him to live there and embraced what the existential psychiatrist J.H. van den Berg called the "different existence" of psychosis.[14] The delusional ideas he developed seemed real, he said, because they came to him in the same way that his mathematical ideas came to him.[15] To Nash, this grandiosity and paranoia, the hallmarks of his psychosis, probably felt like good trade-offs for what Laing would call his "unlivable situation."

Once he had shrugged off the worst of his illness, Nash could acknowledge: "I thought I was a Messianic godlike figure with secret ideas. I became a person of delusionally influenced thinking but of relatively moderate behavior and thus tended to avoid hospitalization and the direct attention of psychiatrists."[16] Nash seems to be saying here that by this time he could distinguish the rational world from the strongly psychotic one he was emerging from. To a considerable degree, he could pick and choose the parts of each world that suited him best.

Nash claims that he partially willed his illness into being and then willed his recovery as well. Of the voices that directed his life while he was seriously ill he said, "I began rejecting them and decided not to listen."[17] His language is direct and strong here, and his words are those of someone who feels he is in control: he "rejected" and he "decided." In 1996 Nash recalled, "I emerged from irrational thinking ultimately, without medicine other than the natural hormonal changes of aging."[18] His decision to live in a rational world was not a one-time thing but, as Nasar points out, a day-to-day recommitment to the consensually validated world: "Nash has compared rationality to dieting, implying a constant, conscious struggle. It is a matter of policing one's thoughts, he has said, trying to recognize paranoid ideas and rejecting them, just the way someone who wants to lose weight has to decide consciously to avoid fats or sweets."[19] Nash's relatively good outcome again reminds us of how heterogeneous the mental illness we call schizophrenia really is. Among other, mostly unknowable, factors an act of Nash's will brought him back from a psychosis he had (at least partly) willed himself into in the first place.

Though the *DSM-IV* is silent on the possibility of a willed contribution to psychotic symptoms, the *DSM-II* (1968) was not fully dismissive of this notion in its attempt to describe schizophrenia: "Disturbances in thinking are marked by alterations of concept formation which may lead to misinterpretation of reality and sometimes to delusions and hallucinations, which frequently appear psychologically self-protective."[20] In *Brave New Brain*, Nancy C. Andreasen, commenting on the changes in the next edition of the *DSM*, admits that "the definition of schizophrenia became more reliable in the new DSM-III criteria, but the essence of its concept may have been lost in the process."[21] Andreasen seems to accept the loss to psychiatry caused by this trade-off, where the purpose of research is served at the expense of the patient.

Taken at face value, John Nash's story challenges some of biological psychiatry's basic tenets about the provenance of delusions and hallucinations. How could a psychotic illness lasting decades, one that clearly makes the *DSM-IV* criteria for paranoid schizophrenia, be willed? Wouldn't a psychosis of that depth and duration have to be a primary brain disease, driven by a chemical imbalance? The fact that an antipsychotic drug sometimes alleviates psychotic symptoms does not mean that the cause of these symptoms is a brain lesion that is directly remediated by the drug. It could be argued that antipsychotic drugs act nonspecifically—involving different brain regions, neurotransmitters, and receptors—to ultimately help patients undercut the distortion of consciousness involved in the original willing into being of their psychotic symptoms. We owe it to ourselves as clinicians, and to our patients, to ask, Do we *need* a "chemical imbalance" to explain a particular psychotic production? If the patient's narrative of life events suggests certain psychodynamic forces (defenses) that are consistent with the symptoms observed, these defenses may be sufficient to explain the patient's psychotic behavior.

It should not be forgotten that the concept of psychosis is a construct that was created to name a way of thinking, feeling, and acting that is significantly different from what is understood as "normal," or, as it is often said, "consensually validated." Consensual validation is a term covering the multitude of ways that "normal" people have agreed to do things. In a dimensional model of mental illness, the line between what is declared "normal" and what is defined as "psychotic" can be seen as being determined by a person's need to continue his life under different rules than the rest of us have chosen to follow, explicitly or implicitly. If a person can construct his world within the "normal" spectrum of consensually validated behavior, who is to say that he is not capable of doing so in the "psychotic" domain as well?

Because psychotic symptoms occur along with certain electrolyte, endocrine, and metabolic derangements, and with the use of some illicit and prescription drugs—all involving real brain "chemical imbalances" and sometimes structural damage—there is no reason to conclude that all psychotic symptoms are caused by changes in brain substrate. Such a false conflation of the provenance of certain kinds of symptoms has resulted in many persons who sought help from mental health professionals becoming patients with mental disorders they never had.

It has been suggested by Laing and others that psychotic behavior can be part of a strategy to ward off anxiety so overwhelming that it radically threatens one's existence.[22] An auditory hallucination could originate as a willed, defensive response of a despairing person to an intolerable situation, a last-ditch effort to shore up a crumbling identity. This process, which would be a psychogenic, functional, psychodynamic, and dimensional phenomenon, could be thought of as a pathological exaggeration of the need many children feel to create imaginary friends and incorporate these fictional characters into their lives.

A cognitive-behavioral model for the treatment of auditory hallucinations has been proposed that includes this explanation for how voices originate: "[H]allucinatory experiences occur when an individual fails to attribute internal, mental events to the self and instead attributes these events to sources that are alien or external to the self."[23] In therapy, patients are taught to "reattribute those voices to themselves" rather than to an external power as they do when they are psychotic.

The American poet Louise Bogan (1897–1970), who experienced her own depressions and mental breakdowns, looked into herself and outward to those she knew and decided that

> All those odd things [people] do, like falling in love with shoes and sewing buttons on themselves and hearing voices, and thinking themselves Napoleon, are natural: have a place. Madness and aberration are not only parts of the whole tremendous setup, but also (I have come to believe) important parts. Life trying new ways out and around and through.[24]

Literary artists have always gone for a larger view of the human enterprise. Bogan's words cut to the heart of what many people who are diagnosed with and treated for a mental illness are trying to accomplish by thinking, feeling, and acting as they do. It has been said that the struggle in any marriage is over who gets to be crazy, or crazier, as the case may be.[25] All behavior has meaning, and pathological behavior has a *different* meaning, which serves a *purpose*. Jean-Paul Sartre, R.D. Laing, Alfred Adler, Gregory Bateson, J.H. van den Berg, and others independently came to this conclusion.

With an artist's intuition, Louise Bogan tried to show us that mental illness is often a way people, who have found it too difficult to live in the "normal" way, choose to live their lives "out and around and through" the problem. If we can learn this lesson, we stand a better chance of helping patients move on to better things. If the lesson is ignored, they may, with our "help," move on to worse things.

CHAPTER 8

How Psychiatry Does Depression Wrong

In the hope of bolstering a "broken brain" theory of depression, and of justifying the use of antidepressants in combating this alleged brain disease, biological psychiatry has proposed an analogy between depression and diabetes. In Type 1 diabetes, the physiological defect has been shown to be a deficiency of insulin caused by autoimmune destruction of the islet β-cells in the pancreas. This deficit is managed, though not permanently overcome, when externally administered insulin lowers high blood glucose, decreasing the insult to the vascular system responsible for the systemic effects of this disease. With diabetes, a physiological disorder of known etiology is targeted with a drug that blunts its deleterious effects.

In spite of claims continuously being made to the contrary, no deficiency of serotonin, epinephrine, or any other neurotransmitter has ever been demonstrated to cause depression in the way that a deficiency of insulin is known to cause diabetes.[1] Those who enthusiastically spin some version of the theory that depression is a biological illness acknowledge, often with a wink, that "there's a lot we still don't know." If a subsequent biopsy confirms the diagnosis, a brain scan showing a higher than normal signal that is consistent with a brain tumor can be said to indicate a tumor. But a low intensity signal reflecting a lower than normal glucose metabolism in the positron emission tomography (PET) scan of a depressed patient does not bespeak depression in the same way.[2]

As a part of their plan to "educate" patients, drug companies have been supplying psychiatrists and primary care physicians with plastic cutaway models showing color-coded components of the limbic system, an area deep in the brain that is generally believed to modulate mood. These models are essentially graven images of the mind reduced to a material mass. They are eye-catching, sculpted objects that are kept on doctors' desks in plain sight. Pointing to the amygdala, the hippocampus, and the hypothalamus, doctors tell patients they are depressed because they have a "chemical imbalance" that will not allow these limbic structures to maintain the electrochemical tone required for normal mood.

The efforts of biological psychiatrists to explain depression as a brain illness ultimately founder on the disjunctive gap between the brain—a physical structure—and the mind, which owes its existence to the brain but is not coincident with it. In *The Perspectives of Psychiatry*, Paul R. McHugh and Phillip R. Slavney call attention to this stumbling block in empirical research: "How does the material brain produce a thing such as the self, 'I,' and how does the brain then relate to it? As yet no scientist can connect this perception of the 'I' and its controlling capabilities totally to what is known of brain structure and function."[3]

McHugh and Slavney spell out the consequences to psychiatry of this brain–mind gap: "Thus, in contrast to cardiologists, psychiatrists cannot go directly from knowing the elements of the brain (neurons and synapses) to explaining the conscious experiences that are the essence of mental life."[4] Some empirical studies have been designed to bridge this gap, but none have demonstrated how a brain neural substrate shapes the contents of consciousness, or, alternatively, how human experience becomes imprinted on a neural substrate. The pharmacology that treats diabetes is not required to bridge the brain–mind gap, but the psychopharmacology that treats depression must do so.

Shortly after the attack on the World Trade Center in 2001, Pfizer ran a TV ad with a voice-over offering this mixture of regret and promise: "We wish we could make a medicine to take away the hurt, but in the meantime … " In the meantime, Pfizer was donating millions of dollars to the survivors' relief fund. Subliminally, this ad was asking us to believe that Pfizer, fronted by all that donated money, was working on a cure for the existential pain that followed the September 11 tragedy and, by extension, the pain that comes with any negative experience.

At the end of 2001, a pharmaceutical analyst interviewed on MSNBC spoke glowingly of new antidepressants in development that were anticipated to be safer than those currently in use. So safe, he claimed, that these drugs could be used to treat patients who have only an occasional down day, or even just the "blues." One of Big Pharma's dirty secrets is that if it is to succeed at the level demanded by executives and stockholders, pharmaceuticals must be sold to people who do not need them.

It does not take long for the fault lines in a culture to be recognized by its artists. In his highly praised novel *The Corrections*, published in 2001,

Jonathan Franzen has Enid Lambert, who at this point in the story is on a cruise with her husband, consult the ship's doctor about her anxiety and sleep disturbance. Enid tries to explain that she is being overwhelmed by the toll that her husband's rapidly advancing Parkinson's disease and dementia is taking on her. But Dr. Hibbard is not interested in listening to Enid's story, and makes it clear that he believes her narrative is irrelevant to her problem. He gives her a new drug, Aslan, which is not yet available in the United States. Though Enid, a conservative, Midwestern, church-going grandmother, has said nothing about feeling ashamed, Dr. Hibbard is certain that her problem is caused by an excess of Factor 28A, the "deep shame" factor, in her brain.

> What's happening at the molecular level, Edna [he's got her name wrong], when you drink those martinis [Enid does not drink martinis], is that the ethanol interferes with the reception of excess Factor 28A, i.e., the "deep" or "morbid" shame factor. But the 28A is not metabolized or properly reabsorbed at the receptor site. It's kept in temporary unstable storage at the transmitter site. So when the ethanol wears off, the receptor is *flooded* with 28A. Fear of humiliation and the craving for humiliation are closely linked: psychologists know it, Russian novelists know it. And this turns out to be not only "true," but *really* true. True at the molecular level. Anyway, Aslan's effect on the chemistry of shame is entirely different from a martini's. We're talking complete annihilation of the 28A molecules. Aslan's a fierce predator.[5]

So much for Dr. Hibbard's grasp of Enid's depression and anxiety. This is his diagnosis and treatment plan.

> Based on your clinical responses I've diagnosed subclinical dysthymia with no observable dementia, and I'm providing you, free of charge [not quite: Dr. Hibbard will soon get his one-hundred-fifty-dollar fee], with eight SampLpacks of Aslan "Cruiser," each containing three thirty-milligram capsules, so that you may comfortably enjoy the remainder of your cruise and afterward follow the recommended thirty-twenty-ten step-down program.[6]

Dr. Hibbard explains to Enid what is pharmacologically unique about Aslan "Cruiser" (she is, after all, on a cruise).

> Mainly, that it switches your anxiety to the Off position. Turns that little dial right down to zero. Aslan "Basic" [another formulation of the drug] won't do that, because to function day to day a moderate

> anxiety level is desirable. I'm on "basic" right now, for example, because I'm working.[7]

Dr. Hibbard's pitch here is just a half-tone up from the patter of the pharmaceutical companies' print and TV advertising. Worse, his words are only a slight parody of what psychiatrists and primary care physicians say to their patients every day.

In 1993, Peter D. Kramer published a book that quickly became a publishing phenomenon. *Listening to Prozac* was Kramer's account of his patients' responses to a new class of antidepressant drug, the selective serotonin reuptake inhibitor, SSRI for short. His subtitle, *A Psychiatrist Explores Antidepressant Drugs and the Remaking of the Self*, gave a good idea of what Kramer was about to claim for Prozac. Prozac was for patients who were severely depressed, but it could also help people who were not really depressed, just unhappy about their lives. Personalities lacking desirable traits could be "remade" with this drug.[8] According to Kramer, after taking Prozac, those who were shy became outgoing. Those who were fearful lost their fears. Those who lacked courage found it in Prozac.

Prozac was doing things that no other drug seemed to have done before. And it was safer than the tricyclic antidepressants (TCAs), which could be hard on the heart and lethal in overdose. Overall, Prozac was said to have fewer and more tolerable side effects than the TCAs. By 1999, 12 years after the green-and-yellow pill came to market, Eli Lilly's Prozac was the third-best-selling drug in the United States.

In 2000, the psychiatrist Joseph Glenmullen, who had worked with many patients medicated with Prozac and the other SSRIs that came later from competing pharmaceutical companies, responded to Kramer's plaudits for this new transformative drug. *Prozac Backlash: Overcoming the Dangers of Prozac, Zoloft, Paxil, and Other Antidepressants with Safe, Effective Alternatives* had a very different story to tell. Many who took SSRIs discovered that the price for "remaking the self," as Kramer had put it in his subtitle, was high, or that the results of this transformation were tinged with a painful irony.

The side effects of Prozac and other SSRIs turned out to be far greater than Kramer had led his readers to believe (to be fair, it takes several years for the side-effect story of any drug to be written). Many users reported feeling numbed by the drugs: "I don't feel like myself" and "I feel like a Zombie" were common complaints. These people were surely not feeling "better than well," though for some who felt bad enough to begin with, feeling numb may have seemed like an improvement. Both men and women told stories about being unable to experience orgasm while taking SSRIs. Many decided that was too high a price to pay and discontinued the drugs. Severe gastrointestinal symptoms, though temporary in some patients, forced others to stop this medication.

A number of patients reported feeling anxious and agitated soon after starting an SSRI. Some said they felt like they were jumping out of their skin. This uncomfortable sensation, known as akathisia, is experienced by many patients who take neuroleptic drugs. Akathisia from SSRIs is believed to have pushed patients to suicide. Some adults who took SSRIs had suicidal feelings they did not have before starting the drug. And then there were those patients who developed muscle twitching and facial tics, which ranged in severity from annoying to disfiguring, and sometimes appeared only after the drug was tapered or withdrawn. This is by no means a complete account of the problems experienced by patients who took SSRIs.[9]

Glenmullen makes a strong case that antidepressants do not specifically target depression-causing chemical imbalances in the brain, but work more generally as psychostimulants and psychoanalgesics. These drugs may indirectly enhance mood and dull pain by strengthening dopamine circuits that underlie the reward response, the same circuits that amphetamine, cocaine, and nicotine act on directly. Before TCAs and SSRIs came to market prescription doses of amphetamine and cocaine were used to treat depression. Glenmullen offers this explanation for how stimulants—and antidepressants—work.

> Except in particularly sensitive individuals, *at prescription doses* all stimulants have similar effects: heightening energy, focusing attention, and brightening mood. As a result, prescription doses are calming even though the drugs are "stimulants." The energizing, mood-brightening, calming, and attention-focusing effects of stimulants have been demonstrated in repeated studies of normal, healthy volunteers.[10]

Like amphetamines, Prozac reduces appetite and promotes weight loss. Many of the side effects and discontinuation effects of SSRIs are the same as those seen with amphetamines.

After lowering the dose of an SSRI, or after quickly withdrawing some SSRIs, symptoms of depression and anxiety sometimes reappear. Often, the prescribing physician interprets this resurgence of symptoms as a sign that the SSRI was working. The patient is then told that the drug needs to be restarted, and possibly taken at a higher dose. These rebound symptoms, collectively called the discontinuation syndrome,[11] are likely the result of a real chemical imbalance that is caused by the SSRI itself, or by a perturbation of brain activity associated with its partial or full withdrawal. Ironically, depressed patients who did not have the chemical imbalance that biological psychiatry insists was the cause of their depression may develop one while taking an antidepressant, or after stopping it.

Besides depression, SSRIs—which, in addition to Prozac, include Paxil, Zoloft, Luvox, Celexa, and Lexapro—have been reported to reduce symptoms of other mental disorders, including social anxiety disorder, phobias, obsessive-compulsive disorder, post-traumatic stress disorder, eating disorders, and sexual addiction. Eli Lilly markets a formulation of fluoxitine hydrochloride (the chemical name for Prozac) called Sarafem, made especially for premenstrual syndrome (PMS). Lilly's Web page for Sarafem advises women that the pink-and-lavender capsules would help them to be "More like the Woman you are," a less boastful variant of the original Prozac hype promising that users will feel "better than well." The efficacy of SSRIs in relieving such a wide spectrum of symptoms is consistent with the idea that these drugs are acting generally as stimulants, rather than as specific antidotes to disparate mental and medical disorders.

An argument frequently heard against the SSRI-as-stimulant theory is that stimulants produce their effect quickly, whereas SSRIs take at least two or three weeks to work as antidepressants. If neuroscience has learned anything about how brain neural networks work, it is that neurons using different neurotransmitters interact, or synapse, with each other. The antidepressant effect of SSRIs may kick in only after increased neurotransmission in serotonin circuits from serotonin-boosting drugs is later coupled with an increase in neurotransmission in synaptically connected dopamine circuits, the principal modulators of stimulus and reward.

The fact that SSRIs meliorate vastly different kinds of symptoms may ultimately be due to the boosting of dopamine circuits that modulate a variety of mental and physical processes. An increased sense of well-being produced by these drugs would reduce anxiety and the need for patients to use defenses underlying many mental disorders. The boosting of dopamine by Zyban, which is the same drug (bupropion) as the antidepressant Wellbutrin, is credited with cutting nicotine craving in cigarette smokers.

Even as patients struggle with the side effects of antidepressants and clinical trials raise questions about the overall efficacy of these drugs, biological psychiatrists continue to use antidepressants as the first-line treatment for depression. When Zoloft was compared with aerobic exercise in a Duke University study of moderately depressed patients, both groups showed equal improvement after four months. After ten months, the exercise group fared better.[12] In some trials, psychotherapy was found to be as effective in treating depression as SSRIs, TCAs, and several newer antidepressants.[13] Other trials have shown that antidepressants were only slightly more effective than placebo, a pill with no active ingredient.[14] If a patient wants a drug—any drug—to work, it may work for the wishing.

My clinical experience has taught me that many people develop symptoms of depression in the first place because they lack sufficient reasons and willpower *not* to develop these symptoms.

There are depressed patients who cannot, or will not, do physical exercise. There are patients who refuse to overcome issues that hold them in a disturbed relationship with the world that is intrinsically depressing. There are patients whose depression is so severe and debilitating that the side effects of medication would not significantly add to their burden. There are depressed patients who are at high risk for suicide. In these instances, antidepressants may be the best first-line treatment.

On the other hand, while taking medication, some of these patients will no doubt be conserving—instead of acknowledging and trying to overcome—a disturbed, and possibly inauthentic, relationship with the world that is *itself* the cause of their depression.[15] In effect, they will be surrendering their freedom to an alleged—and unproven—disturbance in limbic neural tone. At the same time, the sickness of a deteriorating society, which is increasingly unable to support the authentic life of its citizens and inclines many of them toward depression, will also be conserved, effectively guaranteeing Big Pharma an expanding market for its products.

CHAPTER 9
Saving Psychiatry From the Brain

Dr. Benjamin Carson, the renowned director of pediatric neurosurgery at Johns Hopkins Children's Center, did not have the most auspicious start in life. He grew up in what he calls "dire poverty" in Detroit and Boston. His mother could not read. He had low self-esteem, and he did poorly in school. Frequent angry outbursts got him in trouble. Then Carson came across some drawings of the human brain. The incipient neurosurgeon's mind grasped the significance of the fact that, unlike animals, people have frontal lobes. He began to understand what it means to be human.

> Animals are victims of circumstance. They can only react to their environment. But humans, thanks to our frontal lobes, can plan, strategize and exercise control over our environments. We don't have to be victims who simply react.
>
> I learned that truth about frontal lobes at age 10, when—not doing well in school and guided initially by my mother's firm hand—I made a decision to change my life's direction. Within a year and a half, by devouring book after book, I had migrated from the bottom of my fifth-grade class to the top of my seventh-grade class. This academic transformation was so dramatic that one might have suspected a brain transplant, if such a thing were possible. The actual change occurred in my self-perception and my expectations. I had gone from victim to master planner.[1]

Carson's epiphany here is that the human brain subsumes a mind that is largely free to choose its own destiny. His insight, put into action through the power of will, allowed him to go from an urban ghetto to the pinnacle of academic medicine. A careful parsing of Carson's text yields a working model for understanding why so many people become mentally ill: they choose *not* to overcome the obstacles that fate put in their way, or that they themselves created, by refusing the gift of freedom bestowed on them by an evolved human brain. Denying their freedom—often becoming passive in the face of their situation—they make self-deceiving, pathological choices.

Carson's intuition about what the frontal lobes of his brain made possible amounted to a life-transforming experience of personal freedom. It was similar in kind to the epiphany experienced by Jean-Paul Sartre's Roquentin, as he stared at the root of a chestnut tree: "*I exist*, I am the one who keeps it up."[2] Carson's intuition came through a rudimentary understanding of how the human brain works as compared with an animal's brain. Roquentin's intuition did not depend on his understanding of brain neural function, but came directly from his imagining how he could go from a condition of pathological nonfreedom to a freer and happier life. Both Carson and Roquentin were having existential crises at the time of their respective breakthroughs: Carson was failing in school, and his anger threatened to explode into violence; Roquentin had lost himself in his work, and his life was painfully numb.

Most people never reach the degree of transparency about their freedom that Carson and Roquentin did. Unaware of being free, they nonetheless routinely use their freedom to choose between the possibilities that life offers them. When the consequences of some decision are not entirely satisfactory, people will often claim that they had "no choice" but to make that decision. What they are really saying is that the choice not made—the other possibility—would have been even more difficult to make, or harder to live with. Moving unreflectively through one day after another, we often use our freedom, without realizing it, to choose what amounts to the lesser of two evils. It is not surprising that being free does not always *seem* like being free.

That we habitually fail to see how we choose even the most ordinary aspects of our lives sets us up for the illusion fostered by biological psychiatry that our brain—and not *we*—controls our destiny. When psychiatry lost the mind, every problematic thought, feeling, and act became a mental disorder that derived from a malfunction of the brain. In this process, the distinction between what is existential in our struggle to become ourselves (the inherent difficulty) and what is pathological (self-deceiving ways of skirting this difficulty) was obliterated. This is one reason for the "definitional creep" that is becoming increasingly common in psychiatric diagnosis. George E. Vaillant, professor of psychiatry at Harvard Medical School, has noted that "one resident's borderline is another resident's spouse."[3] People have different degrees of tolerance for annoying behavior. Labeling what we find annoying is one way to punish those who annoy us.

When biological psychiatry decided that the mind lacked the power to create a mental illness, it also took away the power of the mind to heal itself. If the brain was sick, it needed a "brain doctor." Henceforth, drugs would be the response to all psychiatric symptoms. There was no need to consider what symptoms meant, because meaning can only come from the mind, and the mind had been pushed out of the picture. When the power once attributed to the mind flowed to the brain, it flowed at the same time from the patient to the doctor who would treat the "broken brain" with drugs. Empowering intuitions of freedom like those experienced by Benjamin Carson and Roquentin became superfluous.

If one sides with Carson and Roquentin in their belief that human freedom is expressed through the mind's power to imagine something beyond the existing state of things, then it follows that this same freedom can be expressed in pathological thinking, feeling, and behavior. Why should freedom be limited to its "normal" expression, and denied pathological expression?

A psychiatric diagnosis is the only diagnosis in medicine that can ultimately be faked. There are no objective tests to diagnose a mental disorder that is not the direct result of a verifiable medical condition. In an article that appeared in *Science* in 1973, David L. Rosenhan, a professor of psychology and law at Stanford University, reported the results of a study designed to see if subjects who were faking symptoms could get themselves admitted to psychiatric hospitals. The article was titled "On Being Sane in Insane Places."[4] Eight "sane" pseudopatients, including three psychologists, a pediatrician, a psychiatrist, a psychology graduate student, a painter, and a housewife, were admitted to 12 different hospitals. Each was hospitalized for between 7 and 52 days. The pseudopatients were prescribed a total of nearly 2,100 pills, including Elavil, Stelazine, Compazine, and Thorazine. Most of these pills were either pocketed or thrown into the toilet—only two were swallowed. All but one pseudopatient was admitted with a diagnosis of schizophrenia, and all were discharged with that diagnosis, and said to be "in remission." No one was outed.

At the time the study was done, psychiatric diagnosis was made with the *DSM-II*. That was before the *DSM-III* introduced what is now claimed to be a more "reliable"—or reproducible—standard for diagnosing mental disorders. (The question of whether the *DSM-IV* allows for a more valid—or accurate—diagnosis is still hotly debated.) Based on my own experience of admitting patients to psychiatric hospitals I would wager that Rosenhan's pseudopatients would not find it any harder now to get admitted under the *DSM-IV*. Depending on the clinician doing the evaluation, besides the symptoms they reported they might have to also claim to be suicidal, homicidal, or both. Under managed care, their stay in the hospital would be much shorter. Of course, they would be given at least as many pills as Rosenhan's proxies, but these would be the newer medications. No wonder the French claim that the more things change, the more they stay the same.

Rosenhan's study demonstrates how vulnerable psychiatrists are to patients who confabulate symptoms of mental illness. It is easy for patients to present themselves as they wish to be seen to clinicians who are willing to see them in that way. This fact should alert us to the ease with which a patient may also deceive *himself* about his thinking, feeling, and behavior, with the intention of creating a psychopathological style that fills his needs and advances his life project. The mind is at work here, and a primary brain malfunction need not be presumed. At least as far back as Freud, patients have been credited with the ability to choose their own mental illness. This is what happened with Adam (Chapter 6) and with Mrs. K (Chapter 7).

Many people who have been diagnosed with mental disorders or who abuse drugs and alcohol can be understood to have made a deliberate and sustained choice—though not necessarily a fully and continuously conscious choice—to live by a different set of rules. Like Adam, who was wrongly diagnosed with schizophrenia, they both knew and didn't know what they were doing. Of course, the mental health profession has its own way of dealing with those who live by special rules that lead to pathology covered by the *DSM*. When patients play their games, clinicians are ready to play their own games in response. This is what we need to learn from Rosenhan's study and from the stories already told here about Adam, Alicia, and others.

Having entertained the suggestion that art, especially literary art, may have more to tell us about mental illness than brain science, it is a small step to accusing biological psychiatry of closing itself off from the best of what has been thought and written in Western culture. One might think that psychiatrists would be the wisest people around, have the best insights into the state of being human, be able to see through the conceits of this world, and help their patients do the same. The word psychiatrist is derived from the Greek: *psyche* = mind; *iatros* = healer. But those who are supposed to be the ultimate experts on healing the mind *reject* the mind, instead of healing it. The psychiatrist now pushes pills on a "broken brain." That is what psychiatrists are expected to do and what they are paid to do.

A kind of religious zeal attaches to the idea that, after centuries of being in the dark about the etiology of mental illness, biological psychiatry has come to rescue patients from their own culpability. That was the point Nancy C. Andreasen hoped to make when she titled her 2001 book about biological psychiatry *Brave New Brain*. The allusion is to Shakespeare's play *The Tempest*: "O, wonder! / How many goodly creatures are there here! / How beauteous mankind is! O brave new world, / That has such people in it!"[5] Now that the brain is to blame for mental illness, it has become a "brave new world" to be explored. Shakespeare intended for those exclamation points to praise a world where the mind still called the shots. But in biological psychiatry, the exclamations are for a brain that, after a certain point in its development, is seen as an autonomous source of mental illness. What is left of the mind now is mostly the domain of clinicians and writers who are not psychiatrists, and those who write self-help books.

We have lost at least a generation of psychiatrists to the illusion of biological psychiatry—often ironically dubbed a "revolution"—which is a monster that is eating the mental health profession alive, ensnaring both clinicians and consumers. Patients need to be saved from psychiatry, and psychiatry needs to be saved from itself. As our mindless society increasingly progresses toward a greedy dystopia, Big Pharma feigns a rescue by coming up with one drug after another to counter the psychiatric symptoms spawned by this social decay—all the while itself becoming a more prominent part of the problem.

To the stories already recounted here demonstrating how the rejection of the concepts of mind and free will has rendered psychiatry a dangerous force, I will add this story about a woman I evaluated in the ER. Jill, who was 47 years old, was brought to the ER by her sister, with whom she lived. Several hours earlier, she had been discharged from a psychiatric hospital after a week's stay. The sister told the triage nurse that Jill was worse when she came out of the hospital than when she went in: she did not seem to understand what was going on around her and reported seeing grass growing on her feet.

Jill had been hospitalized after telling her therapist that she heard a voice instructing her to kill her sister's children. A year earlier, she had been admitted to a state psychiatric hospital for depression and thoughts of harming herself. This was Jill's first brush with the mental health system, and she was diagnosed with bipolar disorder. After discharge, she lived with her sister and the sister's two children, was followed at a community mental health center and took prescribed medication.

During our interview, Jill could not give a straight answer to even simple questions. She looked at the wall in front of her, and asked, "Is that a spot?" She was pointing to something that appeared to be moving. I took this to be a visual hallucination. Jill had no fever, a negative toxicology screen, and a clean urinalysis. All blood counts and electrolytes were within normal limits, and she was not dehydrated. There was no history of hypothyroidism. Jill was delirious, though nothing in her medical workup gave a hint as to why. Her gait was slow and unsteady, and her other movements were indecisive. It was all she could do to draw a lopsided circle on a piece of standard copier paper. Even after several attempts, she could not add to the circle the numbers 1 through 12, as they appear on the face of a clock.[6] This is the first part of the "clock text" used for diagnosing delirium. Jill failed that test decisively.

After ruling out the causes of delirium that would be flagged by abnormalities in the standard ER laboratory tests, I did not have to look far for the reasons behind Jill's confusion and disturbed perception. The community mental health center, where she had been followed for one year, had prescribed Quetiapine, Cogentin, Klonopin, Wellbutrin, Lexapro, Ambien, and Vistaril. Then Geodon, Seroquel, Depakote, and Trazodone were added at the hospital that had just discharged her. Jill was also taking Allegra for bad itching from the Seroquel, prednisone for arthritis, and Hurricaine Gel, a topical anesthetic.

Who could begin to know what this combination of 11 psychotropic medications and 3 somatic medications might do to one patient? (It is hard to know what *one* medication will do to a patient.) I had no doubt that this exercise in polypharmacy was behind Jill's delirium. Her sister agreed: "I just don't want this to happen to anyone else," she told me over the phone after reading the names and dosages of the drugs that had just been added.

Emergency room attending physicians often fail to recognize delirium in psychiatric patients, seeing their change in mental status as a psychiatric, not a medical, problem. Psychiatrists almost never recognize delirium. I have evaluated many delirious ER patients and was successful in getting every one of them admitted to a medical bed for treatment. But not Jill. Because her delirium was judged to be caused by psychotropic medication, it was decided she should go to a psychiatric hospital for a "medication adjustment."

At the time I evaluated her, Jill's psychiatric care could be summarized as a one-year concatenation of errors: misread symptoms led to a misdiagnosis and overmedication led to delirium. To recall a term introduced by Paul R. McHugh, professor of psychiatry at the Johns Hopkins University School of Medicine, Jill had had a "psychiatric misadventure."[7] Her psychiatrists treated her as if she were a mindless brain. The diagnosis of bipolar disorder made during her first hospitalization was almost certainly invalid—both Jill and her sister convinced me that she had never been hypomanic or manic. Jill was constantly depressed, but none of her clinicians ever asked *why* she was depressed. Her depression peaked, and the suicidal thoughts appeared, one year before I saw her in the ER, shortly after her father died (her mother had died several years earlier). Jill told me that her father had molested her when she was 12 years old, and the sister corroborated her story. It seems likely that the father's death had poked a hole in an emotional dike that held her feelings about the abuse in check for over 30 years.

Even in her delirious state, Jill convinced me that the "voice" instructing her to kill her niece and nephew was not a true auditory hallucination, but an internalized thought, which she rejected. At the time she was hospitalized Jill was seriously depressed, and she was not dealing effectively with the recently reopened wounds of her sexual abuse. With the circumstances that forced her to live under her sister's roof, it is no surprise that she would deteriorate emotionally when her niece and nephew got out of hand. Jill made it clear to me that, in spite of what the "voice" said, she did not intend to harm these children, had no plan to harm them, and no means of harming them. Jill's second hospitalization could probably have been avoided had her clinicians bothered to listen to her story, and help her work through what she was feeling.

I called the psychiatrist who had just discharged Jill from the hospital. He had not recognized her delirium. He wanted me to understand that he had 15 discharges that day—some under pressure, no doubt, from managed care. I told him I believed the sexual abuse by Jill's father had been the driving force behind her depression and acute decompensation, and that the father's death one year earlier had triggered the depression. The doctor told me he felt that what had happened 35 years earlier was too remote to be affecting Jill now!

I could only wonder what this psychiatrist had learned during his residency. Like most psychiatrists of his generation, he was probably taught that there are symptoms, chemical imbalances, and medications that correct these imbalances, nullifying symptoms. To me, what happened to Jill and to the other patients whose stories are told here is proof that, unless a clinician knows the dynamic workings of the mind, he will not know how to medicate the brain.

Jill's experience was a reduction *ad absurdum*—the disproof of a proposition by showing the absurdity of its inevitable conclusion—of biological psychiatry's "brave new brain." Her psychiatrist lacked the slightest clue that he had missed the meaning of her initial symptoms, as well as the clear indications of a biological derangement that he himself had caused. In a better world than the one that gave us the current paradigm of biological psychiatry, what happened to Jill would be malpractice. Tragically, it is the standard of care now.

CHAPTER 10
Doing Psychiatry Right

In his article about the pseudopatients who sought admission to psychiatric hospitals by inventing false stories and false symptoms, Rosenhan offered this explanation for why the actors were misread by the clinicians who evaluated and treated them.

> Whenever the ratio of what is known to what needs to be known approaches zero, we tend to invent "knowledge" and assume that we understand more than we actually do. We seem unable to acknowledge that we simply don't know. The needs for diagnosis and remediation of behavioral and emotional problems are enormous. But rather than acknowledge that we are just embarking on understanding, we continue to label patients "schizophrenic," "manic-depressive," and "insane," as if in these words we had captured the essence of understanding.[1]

Almost certainly, this is the reason the "chemical imbalance" that biological psychiatry proposed to explain most mental disorders had such a wide appeal. It was an explanation people badly *needed*, a deus ex machina—literally, a god made from the machine of necessity. People have always looked for ways to escape responsibility for their actions—the unconscious filled the need for many decades—and the chemical imbalance may be the most attractive escape from personal responsibility ever offered.

Naming an abnormal behavior a mental illness is sufficient to make many people think they understand that behavior. Seeing what clinicians call an abnormal brain scan while someone experiences symptoms of the illness is even more convincing. That the observed difference in brain function may be an associative phenomenon, rather than an essential one, is beside the point. Most brain scans of patients with mental illness are functional magnetic resonance imaging (fMRI) scans that measure blood flow. This flow is proportional to brain electrochemical activity, but does not directly measure that activity. The scanned images are generated with a complex apparatus that uses a powerful magnet, electronic sensors, and a computer, which synthesizes a color-coded image of the brain that is viewed on a monitor. This image represents an empirical reduction of some component of the patient's experience, with a result that is many steps removed from the actual experience. In this kind of experiment, the line between science fact and science fiction is not always clear.

Though the brains of patients with mental illness have been scanned since the mid-1970s—for 30 years at this writing—no structural or functional deficit has revealed itself as the *cause* of any mental disorder. Dr. Steven Hyman, former director of the National Institute of Mental Health, is in a good position to see the big picture: "I think that, with some notable exceptions, the community of scientists was excessively optimistic about how quickly imaging would have an impact on psychiatry. In their enthusiasm, people forgot that the human brain is the most complex object in the history of human inquiry, and it's not at all easy to see what's going wrong."[2]

Research in biological psychiatry has provided numerous fragments of knowledge about brain structure and function. A mountain of empirical data has arisen, and contradictory results speak in a multitude of tongues. This outcome is analogous to the result that would be expected if several blindfolded people, who had never seen an elephant, were asked to touch the animal with the intention of determining what the elephant looked like. One blindfolded person would reach out and touch a leg and be convinced the elephant has the shape of a leg; another would reach higher and touch a flank; another would move toward the front of the animal and touch a trunk. Each would be convinced that the elephant had the shape of the part he touched. No one would have touched the whole animal and no one could tell from his empirical experience what the elephant really looked like. Yet each person would believe that he had discovered the truth about the elephant's appearance.

The "blindfold" in empirical psychiatric research is woven from two kinds of fabric: first, the human brain is far more complex than any model so far constructed to explain it, to say nothing of the fact that no two brains, healthy or disordered, are exactly alike; second, whatever it is that allows a material brain to make possible the immaterial functions of the mind remains impervious to empirical investigation. The many published articles and books on the brain and consciousness offer little real information. Much of what is claimed to be known in these publications is expressed at the level of metaphor, and is not literally true. Unfortunately, most of those who write and read these texts do not want to be bothered with this distinction. They would rather believe that they are present at the creation of the "brave new world" of the brain, and will benefit from the "revolution" that biological psychiatry has declared itself to be.

In *The End of Science*, which has the subtitle *Facing the Limits of Knowledge in the Twilight of the Scientific Age*, John Horgan surveyed various theories of consciousness that have been advanced to explain the fact that human beings have material brains, but think, feel, and act in ways that are not ultimately traceable to the activity of this physical mass.[3] The implicit message in most of this work is that whatever mystery is involved in this process, eventually, using the tools of science, it will be solved. Biological psychiatry and Big Pharma have convinced themselves, and try to convince their consumers, that the endless horizon of neuroscience promises all kinds of rewards. Horgan's book calls attention to the unacknowledged limits of these efforts.

Of all the theories about consciousness surveyed by Horgan, the one offered by the British neuroscientist John Eccles seems potentially most useful to psychiatry. Eccles, who won the Nobel Prize for his work on neural transmission in 1963, proposes that the mind exists separately from the brain, even as the brain makes it possible for the mind to function. Eccles's theory is considered "dualistic" because it distinguishes the entities brain and mind.[4] But his idea is actually dialectical because he sees brain and mind as mutually determining one another. The brain allows the mind to choose and to decide.[5] But what the mind chooses and decides in turn influences which brain neurons fire, determining which circuits are formed and strengthened. The neural substrate that is generated as a result of this dialectical process sets into motion and solidifies certain modes of thinking, feeling, or behavior in the developing personality.

Eccles's theory is not deterministic. It allows for the mind, underwritten by the brain, to exercise free will. In this model, we, to a degree, choose our own brain. What we make of our brain becomes an ally or an enemy in the task of constructing our experience moment by moment, choice by choice, following the "*I exist*" imperative that Sartre's Roquentin epitomizes. We can live our lives within the "normal" spectrum of behavior, or outside it. We can "wire" our brains well or badly. Genetics and environment play a part here, sometimes enhancing, sometimes impeding our efforts to respond to the invitation of the world.

In spite of the way biological psychiatry has distorted the meaning of human experience, people are caught up in its magisterium, a word signifying the authority of religious teaching. Even religion is bowing to brain science now. The new discipline of neurotheology has been created to promote the idea that the brain is "wired" to favor religious belief. The limbic system, which includes the amygdala, the hippocampus, and the hypothalamus, is credited with making faith possible. In 2004, *Time* magazine did a cover story on neurotheology,[6] and a book was published on the subject during that year.[7] At the University of Californa Los Angeles Neuropsychiatric Institute, a research team scanned the brains of Democrats and Republicans and concluded that liberals have more active amygdalas than conservatives.[8]

Commenting in *The New York Times Magazine* on a 2005 report about a brain-scan study that appeared in the journal *Nature Neuroscience*, Jim Holt was impressed, but also concerned: "The more that breakthroughs like the recent one in brain-scanning open up the mind to scientific scrutiny, the more we may be pressed to give up comforting metaphysical ideas like interiority, subjectivity and the soul. Let's enjoy them while we can."[9] Holt is naming functions and powers of the mind that biological psychiatry does not recognize. The wisdom about what it means to be human and to have a mind capable of making free choices—accumulated over nearly three millennia by philosophers and nearly two centuries by psychiatry, psychoanalysis, and psychology—seems to be rejected now as much by the consumers of psychiatric services as by those who provide these services.

In 1970, I read R.D. Laing's *The Divided Self*, which is subtitled *An Existential Study in Sanity and Madness*. This book changed my career and my life. Laing had an understanding of both the "normal" and the pathological world that came from his reading of the European existential philosophers, especially Martin Heidegger and Jean-Paul Sartre. Before discovering Laing, I had read Sartre's *Existentialism and Human Emotions*,[10] and been struck by how right his ideas about existence preceding essence, nothingness, nihilation, freedom, contingency, authenticity, self-deception, and facticity felt. But *The Divided Self* was the first text I encountered that explicitly linked these ontological notions with mental illness and its treatment.

I delved into the thinkers who had influenced Laing. Studying at Johns Hopkins with the existential philosopher Ralph Harper,[11] I read, in addition to Sartre and Heidegger, Kierkegaard, Nietzsche, Unamuno, Ortega y Gasset, Camus, Merleau-Ponty, Marcel, and Tillich. I recognized in the texts of these thinkers an implicit therapeutic: their ontology sketched the structure of human Being, emphasizing the fact that behavior is purposeful and has *meaning*. Even before I became a clinician, I inferred that some distorted ontological meanings could take the form of mental illness.

Later, I read the work of European psychiatrists and psychoanalysts, who like Laing, had absorbed the existential tradition and applied it to their clinical work: Ludwig Binswanger, Medard Boss, Karl Jaspers, Viktor Frankl, and J.H. van den Berg.[12] I combined elements of this tradition with biological psychiatry and practiced from an integrated paradigm.

Eventually, I realized that biological psychiatry was failing to help most patients and harming many of them because, in the course of assigning to the brain the primary responsibility for everything a person thinks, feels, and does, the psychological meaning and structure of patients' behavior—the essence of their human Being—was being ignored.

Centuries before psychiatry came to its current crisis, the French psychiatrist Philippe Pinel (1745–1826) understood the tendency of physicians who practice the healing art to overreact: "In diseases of the mind ... it is an art of no little importance to administer medicines properly; but, it is an art of much greater importance and more difficult acquisition to know when to suspend or altogether to omit them."[13] When psychiatry lost the mind and ascribed mental illness to a malfunction of the brain, and "meaningless" symptoms were used to make categorical diagnoses from the *DSM*, a natural inclination of clinicians to overpathologize, overdiagnose, and overmedicate was unleashed.

The power of suggestion is strong in any case, but stronger still when that suggestion is made to a vulnerable patient by a doctor. Patients tend to grow into the shoes of their wrong diagnosis and to become the kind of person their clinicians say they are. Many times, when I doubted the validity of an ER patient's bipolar or schizophrenia diagnosis, I would ask if he believed he had that illness. "That's what my doctor told me," was a common response, made in a tone indicating that the patient implicitly trusted the doctor's call.

One of the implications of the epiphany "*I exist ...*" experienced by Roquentin in Jean-Paul Sartre's novel *Nausea* is that the life we create invariably unfolds and develops as themes in a story. To exist is to create a narrative about ourselves, others, and the world. "The power of narrative is shattering, overwhelming," says the novelist Robert Stone. "We are the stories we believe; we are who we believe we are. All the reasoning of the world cannot set us free from our mythic systems. We live and die by them."[14] As a clinician, I must challenge the claim that nothing can be done to change the power a story has over us, since that is precisely what a good deal of psychotherapy attempts to do.[15]

When I am listening to a patient's story for the first time, I try to determine the level of disturbance the narrative is revealing, or, to put it another way, how deep the psychological "lesion" is.[16] The first issue to be decided is whether the patient's suffering is primarily existential, or pathological. Is he simply stuck on some problem with living that he cannot—or will not—find a way to overcome? If so, I try to show him that this is the problem and convince him that he, like Sartre's Roquentin, has this ability, if he would only accept the implications of the intuition "*I exist ...*"

In his attempt to understand mental illness from the existential perspective, the German psychiatrist Karl Jaspers (1883–1969) defined what he called a "boundary situation."[17] All of us have faced situations where we could not go forward, but could not retreat from either. In effect, we get "stuck" at a line that we cannot cross. Many people fumble and stumble while caught in these situations as they refuse to bear the pain of being stuck and exert the kind of effort it would take to authentically cross the line, and become unstuck. Often psychotherapy amounts to helping the patient cross this boundary, on elbows and knees if that is what it takes. Jaspers's boundary situation is a more profound way of naming the metaphorical space occupied by those who are said to be "caught between a rock and a hard place."

When it becomes clear to me that significant pathological defenses have come into play in a patient's struggle to deal with (or avoid) what challenges him most, I try to determine the severity of these defenses. I find the designations neurotic, borderline, and psychotic useful, though imprecise, as I attempt to conceptualize a patient's pathology dimensionally. To think of mental illness in this way is to infer a continuum of meanings to any behavior, ranging from normal and productive at one end of the spectrum to pathological and destructive at the other. At certain points in the continuum of meanings, behavior becomes increasingly maladaptive: bad for the doer, bad for others, and bad for society. At these points, labels are usually attached and diagnoses made. A major advantage of this *dimensional* approach is that it allows for the meaning of a behavior to stay attached to the behavior. When diagnosis is made with the *categorical* approach, relying mostly on the *DSM* checklist of "meaningless" symptoms, this connection is often lost.

Neurotic patients, derogatorily referred to as the "walking wounded," suffer intensely over matters that seem trivial to others. In his films, Woody Allen has done as much as anyone to describe the neurotic personality of our time. Neurotics suffer—and make others suffer—but they usually find a way to stumble along in the world. In spite of their suffering and dysfunction, many are high achievers.

We may laugh at the pains of neurotics, but no one writes comedies about the often self-destructive lives led by those having what Otto F. Kernberg calls borderline personality organization.[18] I chose Kernberg's term over the *DSM*'s borderline personality disorder because this designation is consistent with the dimensional approach to diagnosis. The primitive defenses used by borderline patients often prohibit them from attaining stable associations with "normal" others. Normalcy is a relative concept in any case. But when one sees how borderline patients function, what Freud called the "psychopathology of everyday life" seems rather "normal" in comparison. Few of the more seriously ill borderline patients are high achievers because their pathology does not permit them to make the sustained effort that success demands.

Finally, patients who are genuinely psychotic—and this by no means includes everyone who has been diagnosed with a psychotic disorder—are disturbed to the degree that, temporarily or permanently, they cannot share significant parts of what has been called our "consensually validated" world. This is the everyday world of cause and effect that "normal" people inhabit. Some, but not all, patients who have psychotic symptoms will benefit from antipsychotic medication. It was argued earlier that "psychotic" symptoms can be psychogenic. Antipsychotic medication can help these patients control their symptoms, until the underlying inauthentic constructs are authentically resolved. Those with severe mood swings that seem to owe less to the psychodynamics of a personality disorder than to a primary biochemically induced mood disorder often need a mood stabilizing drug, and sometimes an antipsychotic drug.

Having determined from the patient's story whether his pathology is predominantly neurotic, borderline, or psychotic, I proceed to "unpack" the story, searching for key pathological elements which, when taken together, comprise his illness. I look for telltale signs of self-deception that may be keeping him from playing the cards that life dealt him more productively. I challenge the idea that his handling of a situation in a way that continues to cause him emotional pain was the *only* way he could have handled it—at the time when the choice was initially made, or at any time after that. I try to convince those patients who are strong enough to hear it that many psychiatric problems originate in a refusal to make an authentic response to a significant life challenge, whether this is rooted in early abandonment, a later loss or trauma, a Jasperian boundary situation, or something else.

The most serious psychiatric diagnoses, particularly schizophrenia, are said to be "diagnoses of exclusion." This means that before a diagnosis can be made, lesser diagnoses, representing lesser degrees of pathological distortion, must be ruled out. In fact, every psychiatric diagnosis should be a diagnosis of exclusion. Occam's razor needs to be applied to the elements of each patient's story, and the principle of parsimony applied as a way of limiting a clinician's tendency to overreact and overdiagnose.

There are those who claim that psychiatric diagnosis became more valid after the *DSM-III* was introduced in 1980. My clinical experience does not support this claim. Symptoms that have been shorn of their meaning can be plugged into any number of the *DSM* symptom lists to justify the diagnosis of any number of mental disorders. A valid diagnosis requires the alignment of symptoms and meaning. Nothing in the *DSM-III* and *DSM-IV* guides the clinician in making this match.

Clinicians using the *DSM-IV* often make a diagnosis that does not reflect what is really happening in a patient's life—a result favored by the procrustean bed of a categorical taxonomy based on symptoms of unspecified meaning. To lessen the distortions of the *DSM*'s categorical imperative and open a dimensional axis that gives the meaning and structure of symptoms their due, the diagnosis of someone who's thinking, feeling, and behavior are sufficiently different from the norm to be called a mental disorder should be accompanied by a detailed description of these aberrations. The language of psychiatry should be avoided here, and the words used should capture, as closely as possible, the phenomena constituting the illness. For some patients, this narrative would be the truest diagnosis of all.

When biological psychiatry revoked the mind, it made a generation of patients into neural cripples. These cheated people deserve to have their minds and their freedom restored to them. A new paradigm for psychiatry, if that is in the cards, would have to begin by ensuring that no one else is harmed in this way.

Johns Hopkins psychiatry professor Paul R. McHugh believes that "we labor under a strange classificatory system—one that insists that we define mental disorders by their symptomatic appearance."[19] McHugh is calling for a "new conceptual structure [that] would insist on defining mental disorders by their essential natures rather than by their appearances alone." This is another way of saying that we need to know the meaning of symptoms before a valid diagnosis can be made.

In *The Perspectives of Psychiatry*, McHugh and coauthor Phillip R. Slavney present a plan for bringing about this change. They believe that the paradigm of biological psychiatry, which has all but owned the profession since about 1970, is inadequate and needs to be replaced by a system of classification and diagnosis that is anchored in the "study of life at the psychological level." The new paradigm would seek to understand the brain function that makes psychological life, the life of the mind, possible.

McHugh and Slavney distinguish mental illnesses that are primary brain diseases from those that derive mainly from the conflicts that people experience as they use their freedom to pursue their lives: "Some psychiatric disorders are expressions of nature's power over human life. ... Other psychiatric disorders are expressions of personal distress due to life events."[20] Ultimately, brain and mind are inextricably joined whether a mental illness is rooted primarily in the brain pole or in the mind pole of what can be thought of as a dialectical unity of brain and mind. Adolf Meyer, who was on the psychiatry faculty at Johns Hopkins between 1910 and 1940, coined the term psychobiology to name this dialectic.[21] Meyer's way of doing psychiatry flourished in America during his time at Hopkins. But psychobiology lost out to the influence of Freud and psychoanalysis, which arrived at our shore around 1940 and lasted until about 1970, when the biological "revolution" in psychiatry began. Meyer's work lacked an empirical and systematic foundation, which is one reason why his approach did not stand up to competing ideologies.

By systematizing Meyer's method and bringing in new empirical data, McHugh and Slavney hope to revitalize the Meyerian vision of psychobiology, which, historically, has been one of the most successful efforts to specify the mind–brain dialectic in mental illness. They offer four "perspectives," or ways of seeing how and why a person may be mentally ill:

1. Many illnesses of known etiology that cause changes in mental status are best understood as diseases (Alzheimer's, tertiary syphilis); mental disorders such as schizophrenia and bipolar disorder, which involve neuropathology of unknown etiology and kind, fit the disease model in some, but not all ways.
2. Pathological behavior is dimensional, which is to say it is a diminished or exaggerated variant of normal behavior.
3. Personality styles, whether "normal" or disordered, are the sum total of how we make our lives, facilitated or limited by genetics and development.
4. The stories we tell about ourselves, others, and the world are components of the deep structure of our lives, and can take on pathological meanings that make us mentally ill.

Taken together, the four perspectives give both mind and brain their due. In the effort to understand and address abnormal behavior, clinicians are offered a way to think about what medical science has to contribute and what can come only from the insights of literature, philosophy, psychology, and other humanistic disciplines.

One could imagine using this four-perspective approach, which is sensitive to the meaning of behavior and thus to the meaning of symptoms, to create a classification and diagnostic system that would replace the multi-axial *DSM*.[22] In spite of revisions, the *DSM* is still plagued by the wrongheaded division of Axis I and Axis II disorders, by a categorical, rather than a dimensional understanding of pathological behavior, and by an implicit directive that symptoms of unspecified meaning can be used to diagnose psychiatric illness.

Psychiatry's greatest challenge now is to understand and address the "bottom-up" and "top-down" components of each patient's problem.[23,24]

If a skeletal person can look in a mirror and insist "I'm fat," and then act on that perception by continuing to avoid food in the hope of correcting the situation, the mind would seem to be capable of attributing just about *any* meaning to *anything*. Psychiatry needs to start a large-scale empirical inquiry that would definitively establish the mind's "top-down" capacity—enabled by a complementary "bottom-up" biological substrate—to construct what we think of as normal human experience, along with those outlying thoughts, feelings, and acts called mental illness. This project should be pursued with the same intensity that biological psychiatry brought to the attempt to explain mental illness as a primary chemical imbalance of the brain.

EPILOG

A Man, Crippled by Anxiety, Who Was Previously Misdiagnosed With Bipolar Disorder: Therapy Leading to Structural Change

Many of the criticisms made of biological psychiatry in the preceding text, as well as the prescriptions offered for changing this paradigm, are exemplified in the clinical story that follows.

Peter was referred by his primary care physician. Always anxious, he had recently become more so, and his sleep was down to a few hours each night. Peter's anxiety seemed to keep him from sleeping, and the fact that he could not sleep made him more anxious. In his panic, he was reaching out to friends and relatives. "I'm driving them crazy," he reported, knowing that he could not continue doing so.

Peter was 57 years old and had been retired for 7 years. "Work was too stressful," he said. He lived alone in a house that had been passed on to him after his parents died. His only regular activity was doing volunteer work for a senior citizens center. He had been in the Air Force from age 17 to 19, but was given a general discharge, due to what he called his "bad attitude." Peter earned a bachelor's degree in social science when he was 25, and then took graduate courses in social work part-time while working for the Department of Social Services. He quit that job when he was 30 and received a master's degree in social work the following year. His last employment was a 17-year stint with a foster care agency, where he ultimately became a supervisor. He let it be known that he lasted as long as he did in that job only because his boss had been tolerant of his "short fuse." Peter was nothing if not self-effacing.

At age 19, Peter spent several days in a psychiatric hospital because, as he put it, "I was too argumentative." He took Thorazine during that time, but claims that the drug did nothing for him. Later, while in college, he had 6 months of psychotherapy. He had no further psychiatric care until coming to the private practice group where I worked, more than 30 years later. No one in his family had ever been diagnosed with a mental disorder.

Peter's primary care physician was concerned enough about the headaches Peter reported, along with his anxiety, to order a magnetic resonance imaging (MRI) scan of his brain; no abnormalities were found. Tests for thyroid and liver function, as well as the usual blood work, came back normal. Peter was taking Synthroid for hypothyroidism and Xanax at bedtime to alleviate anxiety and to help with sleep. He had been prescribed Seldane for allergies and sporadically took several over-the-counter drugs for hay fever, insomnia, and nasal congestion. He had a history of elevated blood pressure and cholesterol, but was not being medicated for either condition during the time I saw him.

Believing that Peter's fast talking and tendency to jump quickly from one topic to another were symptoms of hypomania, the psychiatrist from our group who did the initial evaluation and then referred Peter to me for psychotherapy diagnosed bipolar II disorder and generalized anxiety disorder. He was started on Tegretol. Although the many manifestations of his anxiety were Peter's main psychiatric complaint, dysthymia was also a part of his problem. In fact, dysthymia had been Peter's principal mood during most of his life.

From the psychiatrist's chart notes, it was clear that he originally conceived Peter's problem as a brain disorder—bipolar II is generally regarded as such—that should be addressed primarily with Tegretol. In a note from a week before I met with Peter for the first time, the psychiatrist wrote, "Internal referral for psychotherapy made to help patient address dating, etc." In other words, Peter's social isolation, loneliness, and inability to connect with women were to be relegated to psychotherapy while the problems caused by his anxiety and mood lability were to be addressed with pharmaceutical agents. The psychiatrist's note from a few days later read, "Explained potential for improvement will not be demonstrated until he has had a therapeutic blood level of Tegretol at least one week."

I started working with Peter on July 18, 1995. We finished 21 months later, on April 24, 1997. We met 82 times, weekly, until 3 months before termination, then monthly after that.

It is fair to say that we hit the ground running—Peter was 15 minutes early for his first appointment. We were a good therapeutic match from the start. At a very basic human level, we got along. I believe I was able to quickly convince Peter that I had a handle on what was happening in his life, and understood why he was suffering. He always showed up ready to work. For all the anger and verbal outbursts that he reported directing at others, he was never angry at or in any way abusive to me. What might be thought of as the "anxious structures" that made up his life were quickly identified and challenged. It was these structures that we chipped away at, week by week. Our work was ultimately judged to be successful by both of us.

After just a few hours of listening to Peter's story, I had no doubt that he was not, and had never been, hypomanic and that the diagnosis of bipolar II disorder was incorrect. (Peter told me that he had always talked fast.) I was also convinced that his mood lability was not due to a primary mood disorder. The dynamics of his changes in mood were easily traced to an almost constant anger that was rooted in a deep and pervasive anxiety. This angry transformation of his experience kept him from taking the minimal amount of nourishment from the world that is necessary to be a real player there. Peter's ultimate problem was that he was *not* a player, and wanted to be one.

In retrospect, the 21-month course of our work can be divided, if somewhat arbitrarily, into two phases: the free fall that brought Peter to therapy was halted and the first steps forward were taken; then a steady improvement began, which continued until he felt our work was done.

Stabilization and Initial Improvement (5 Months, 23 Meetings)

Typically, a mental status examination reports the degree of "distress" a patient appears to be in at the time. At our first meeting, Peter's distress was not acute enough for him to be seen in an emergency room or to be considered as a candidate for hospitalization. But it was clear that he was in deep pain. His face wore the look of distress. He was jittery. He spoke fast and nervously, as if he was trying to save himself from annihilation, with gushes of words that clearly stated what he was feeling. He jumped from topic to topic, but everything he said made sense. Peter was reaching out to me in the hope that I could save him. Like so many people with the kind of problem he was having, Peter had occasional thoughts that he might be better off dead, but denied any intent or plan to harm himself. Neither he nor anyone in his family had ever made a suicide attempt.

The only recent change in Peter's life was that, 5 weeks before he came to our group for help, he had developed insomnia. He had always been able to nap during the day to escape anxiety or boredom and still sleep 6 to 8 hours at night. Now he had trouble getting to sleep at all. When sleep did come, he woke after an hour or two. As this problem worsened, Peter shared his despair with his primary care physician. After seeing that the Xanax he had prescribed would not do the job, this doctor called for a psychiatric consultation.

"When I lost the ability to sleep," Peter told me, "that's when I panicked. I had a good facility for sleeping when I was bored … I suppressed the *fear* of falling asleep." There it was, at our first meeting, a significant part of his problem, self-revealed, with minimal prompting from me. This was an authentic cry from the depths. The pressure of what he was hiding from—his dissatisfaction with the life he had made—could no longer be held back by sleep. Peter did not trust the world enough to let go of wakefulness and relinquish himself to the ambiguities of a state where he was required to cede control. "I see it as something I have been suppressing for a long time. I feel a sense of hopelessness. My life stinks … Lousy … Nothing to do … I have a wonderful facility for keeping things down."

Like so many persons with severe anxiety, Peter had a long list of somatic complaints, which he described to me during our second hour. Bad, nagging headaches topped the list. These headaches had plagued him for years, but had become particularly bothersome during the previous 5 weeks. Other aches and pains, all over his body, were a constant challenge to his mood and his physical strength. A rash and a low-grade temperature came and went and came again, without diagnosis. Four or five times a year, he could count on being awakened during the night with chest pains, which were relieved by drinking water. My guess was that most of these symptoms were somatic expressions of anxious feelings that Peter has never been able to deal with, and are best understood as components of generalized anxiety, not panic.

Peter kept the insight coming. "I see a hard time changing this," he warned me. "I had many chances to do things and didn't take them. I didn't have confidence in myself. I didn't feel I was attractive to women. When I did have a relationship, I was afraid to keep it going. I was afraid of sex. I had little experience with it." No mask here, and no cover-ups to challenge. Peter was ready to deal, and he knew how hard this was going to be. He was talking about changing the patterns—and emotional structures—of a lifetime.

When Peter was 21, to his surprise, a woman at a summer camp where he was working pursued him. But when she began telling him about the complex emotional tangle that was her family's life, Peter was overwhelmed by this revelation and quit the relationship. "I was afraid to get involved," he told me. For most of his life, Peter was content to be by himself. Now he feels that his life alone has been wasted and wants to reach out to other people and broaden his horizon. But he does not know how. When he tries to make a connection with someone, the anxiety that invariably comes up leads to conflicts he cannot resolve, and he is paralyzed. Such is Peter's dilemma.

Part of my job working with Peter was to encourage him to make contacts that would extend his horizon and let him break out of a shell of isolation that he had hidden in for most of his life. At our fourth meeting, he told me that he had joined the Jewish community center's athletic program and planned to sign up for the singles program as well. "The thought of doing this scares the hell out of me," he said. Peter's anxiety was twofold: he was afraid of making the moves necessary to overcome his isolation and he was afraid that, if he did not make these moves, he would be crushed by the worsening anxiety that brought him to therapy. He implicitly grasped his dilemma.

Negativity, impatience, irritability, worry, and paranoia are some of the components of Peter's pathological style of living. He knows that these traits have kept him from doing what is necessary to satisfy his needs. Throughout his career as a social worker, his "bad" attitude, as he put it, had caused problems with coworkers and led to his early retirement. "I get too easily irritated. I haven't developed an attitude toward other people that is positive. I want things to happen too fast—part of this is the worry 'I can't do it' or 'I won't be successful.' I get mad when I drive and other drivers don't follow the rules." Peter was acknowledging a low tolerance in conflict situations. This was a major factor in what he saw as a largely "wasted" life. "Sometimes my worry borders on paranoia. I can't control it. When the situation is over, I know people weren't doing anything to me. But then it starts again. Even when I say 'You're being paranoid,' I would still have the feelings and it would still bother me. It spoils the enjoyment." At times like this, Peter's thinking and emotions were not in sync. He worried constantly about money even though he knows he had, as he put it, "beaucoup money."

Peter has reported at each meeting the ups and downs in his level of anxiety and mood during the preceding week. At the fifth meeting he volunteered that he had "gone downhill over the weekend." He had more than the usual trouble sleeping, was more anxious and woke up feeling hot and faint. He had a disturbing dream about "a process or procedure that I was not doing right." The dream frightened him and repeated a day or two later. I suspected that the defective "process or procedure" that arose from his subconscious was a dream-work equivalent of his "wasted" life. We were tweaking Peter's defenses when we engaged in our dialogue, and transient flares of increased anxiety were to be expected. "I don't know if I have it in me to do difficult things," was Peter's response to my interpretation. Peter was starting to face issues he had avoided all his life, and this was causing him additional pain, but not more pain than he could handle. The dream came again, the next week. "This is like starting life all over again," he said.

Peter began our eighth meeting by telling me about what he considered a "slip" in his efforts to get better control of his behavior and achieve greater mutuality with others. On the way from his car to my office, while crossing the street, a woman yelled at him and he responded with an obscenity. "I give myself a black mark for that," he said. This incident shows how assiduously Peter is pursuing his rehabilitation. He told me that my help with identifying the main features of his neurotic style—negativity, impatience, irritability, worry, and paranoia—was allowing him to make specific changes in his behavior as he encounters certain situations. I pointed out that every time he does something to challenge one of these neurotic elements, by acting differently than he would have habitually acted, he is internalizing that difference and becoming a little more like the person he aspires to be.

"It will take a year or two to get myself together," Peter told me at the top of our ninth meeting. "This is the situation. I can handle it. I will not fall apart." Peter had already stopped the 5-week free fall that made him seek help. Then, during the next 2 months, he took another step, projecting what he thought of as the "re-creation of myself." We had the same vision for the task ahead: we were working for permanent, structural change.

Peter brought some written notes to this meeting and he read them to me. "I always say 'no' at first when someone makes a suggestion. I'm stubborn. I only do what I want to do. It has to be *my* idea." For as long as he can remember, Peter has been this way. What he was acknowledging here is ultimately a lack of reciprocity with other people and with the world. There is something deficient—and pathological—about his basic stance toward everyone and everything outside himself. This is a part of his style, and underneath that, the structure of his Being. This is what needs to be changed.

During our sixth meeting, Peter made a disclosure that surprised me. "I don't listen well. My mind races on to something else. I pick up the main points, but I don't hear all you say." (I suspect that he was hearing more of what I say than he hears from other people. This kind of attention is necessary for the therapeutic work we are doing.) Somehow, defensively, Peter has learned to turn down the signal of what he hears from others. Perhaps the signal is swamped by the noise that his anxiety has generated between himself and everyone else. The "cocoon" that Peter acknowledges living in for most of his life receives a reduced signal from the outer world.

Peter often reports feeling the knife-edge of heightened anxiety during our meetings. One minute he wonders out loud if he can deal with these uncomfortable feelings. The next minute he assures himself—and me—

that he can. Each time he anxiously goes through a situation more daring than those he has been used to, and then comes out the other end safely, he becomes more convinced that his anxiety is, ultimately, related to how he chooses to deal with others and the world. For as long as it takes to change a style that never worked well for him, and then stopped working altogether, living on an anxious knife-edge is the only way he will authentically and permanently ever get out of that bad place.

During our next few meetings, Peter continued to brood over what he had made of his life. But his disappointment about how things had turned out was partly balanced by his sense that his life would soon be improving. "Is this all there is?" he asked as if not expecting an answer. "Am I going to be able to do more? I don't know what to do except keep going. What's the use of brooding? Analyzing it doesn't make it any better." But later, he said: "I've turned a little corner. Nothing that has happened has thrown me. I feel I'm getting something, learning something." The balance in what Peter says here is tipped toward the future. His words imply forward movement. He shows pride at some small accomplishments and acknowledges that there is really no permanent downside to what he is doing. For someone who has focused on the past and the negative, this is a step up, but not an easy one: "It's so hard to change. How do you do it? Can I do it?" Peter seems to implicitly understand that the answers to these questions can only be found in his moving forward.

Our fourteenth meeting came at the end of a week that Peter described as "miserable." He felt "very discouraged and down." He had slept for only four and a half hours the previous night and woke several times with hot flashes. The following story demonstrates how little it takes to throw Peter off his game—and the kind of problem, in one manifestation or another, that has plagued him all his adult life. He had agreed to participate in a registration drive for senior citizens at the Jewish community center. Then a number of people who volunteered did not show up. Peter realized that he would be required to do more work than he had anticipated. He became frightened at the prospect of being overwhelmed by the drive and stayed away from the center for several days. Looking ahead, these thoughts ran through his mind: "This is going to be too hard for me. I can't do it. Too many things could go wrong. I couldn't handle it."

It took a few days for Peter to resolve this problem, but he did resolve it. He agreed to stay on the registration committee but declined to be the one responsible for the outcome. This was a partial solution, but a solution nonetheless. He smoothed the feathers he had ruffled while the problem was playing out. He had backed off from a chance to take on a higher level of responsibility and commitment than he originally contracted for, but ultimately followed through on what he initially agreed to do. Peter's sleep improved and there were no more hot flashes.

But a new traumatic experience reared its head a few days later. Peter has spoken several times about how much he regrets never becoming significantly involved with *any* woman, in spite of his chances to do so. At our fifteenth meeting, this issue came front and center. A friend offered to introduce Peter to a woman he knew. Peter's anxiety soared. Should he, or shouldn't he, go out on this date? "If I don't do it now," he told me, "I'll never have an opportunity to. I don't want to give up on this one." Peter's anxiety has two parts: first, that his self-imposed cocoon will not be satisfactory to sustain his life, and second, that he is not willing to take the risks necessary to get out of that enclosure. "The possibility of starting the relationship … I don't want the stress, the flushes … In my mind, I can do it … In my gut, I can't." Peter was clearly referring here to the somatic manifestations of his anxiety. When his stress goes up, his body tenses and says, in effect, no to the risk he is considering.

Peter is caught between going for it and running from it. "I can't be alone forever," he said. "I've been in this rut so long. It's like an animal who can't change his habits. Every second I want to give up." But he is not giving up. It is interesting that Peter used the analogy of an animal—a species that lacks the range of freedom humans have—when speaking of the rut he is in. In his head, he feels he should be able to make this move, but his (animal-like) gut holds him back.

At our next meeting, Peter reported the following thought about the possibility of taking up his friend's offer to get him a date: "She will want to live with me and marry me." This rumination presumes a good deal. Arrogance aside, Peter reveals himself here as a world-class catastrophizer: put any play in motion and Armageddon will be the inevitable result. I pointed out to Peter that he hadn't even *met* this woman. His reply: "The thought of doing anything to get involved with someone, taking that step … the *idea* of dating … obsessing about it." Here again is Peter's obsessive loop: I don't have it in me to do it … I should give it up … I should do it.

I asked if he ever had an experience of doing something that caused him as much pain as the pain he suffers *anticipating* a new situation. No, he said thoughtfully. I pointed out how his negative thoughts led to negative behavior (paralysis of his projected project), along with the somatic concomitants of this paralysis, which, in turn, led to negative outcomes (isolation, disappointment, regret)—a vicious cycle if there ever was one. Peter's response? "I'm trying harder than I ever have before. I'm feeling better than ever." If, through all this pain, Peter is *feeling better than ever*, we must be doing something right.

At the top of our seventeenth meeting, Peter reported that things had taken a turn for the worse—again: "Miserable. I'm feeling so God-damned down. I'm sick of not being able to sleep and waking up flushed." Peter spoke at length—a monologue, really—about his agitation and what he might do to change things. I pointed out that since we have been meeting, we have been dealing with emotionally charged issues and that he has made a considerable effort outside our meetings—in the real world—to do things he has not previously done, which are also emotionally charged. All of this expressed emotion is making him feel uncomfortable, as the defenses of a lifetime are tweaked, loosened, reinstated (sometimes less tenaciously) and then loosened again. What Peter and I are really doing is titrating the amount of discomfort he can take as he moves forward and out of his cocoon, into a life that has a better chance of satisfying him.

It was, no doubt, Peter's complaints about the discomfort he was experiencing that led his psychiatrist to prescribe BuSpar. This anti-anxiety drug was added 4 months after we started. Problems with sleep have been one of Peter's chief complaints, and Benadryl, to be taken at bedtime, was also prescribed. Up to this point, my efforts to convince the psychiatrist that Peter was not bipolar had been unsuccessful. The Tegretol, which Peter started taking right after the bipolar diagnosis was made, was continued, but gradually tapered.

"It seems like the BuSpar is doing something," were Peter's opening words at our next meeting. "I'm feeling more optimistic. Not feeling down in the morning." (This was one week after the drug was started; generally, BuSpar has an induction period of several weeks, raising the possibility that he was experiencing a placebo effect). We talked about whether BuSpar was responsible for the changes Peter reported. He reiterated his belief that the Tegretol he had been taking for 4 months did not help him. He doubted that the Benadryl he had just started was doing him any good, either. Why he credited BuSpar and not Benadryl with his improved sleep he did not say. I explained that the ideal situation would be if, as he tries to reach out for more life, BuSpar were to take enough of the edge off the discomfort he feels to encourage him to continue reaching. I thought I sensed a note of resolve I had not previously heard when Peter asked, "Where do I go from here?" He made it sound like he definitely wanted to go somewhere. Then he added, "I want to have a couple of weeks feeling good first."

Five months after we started our work, during our twenty-second meeting, Peter took his own inventory:

"I have a low tolerance for anything physical or mental that makes me feel uncomfortable."

"I never did see how I could overcome it. I always thought of it as being in my genes."

"I make the same mistakes over and over. I want more out of life, but I don't see how I will ever have it. I don't accept that."

"I can't have a relationship with a woman. I can't even take the stress of thinking about it."

This is mostly familiar stuff, but there are at least two interesting revelations here. This was the first time Peter let it be known that he had thought his anxiety was genetic. What is genetic cannot be changed and is, in the current parlance of brain science, "hardwired." (Peter's male-pattern baldness is genetic.) Has 5 months of meeting weekly with someone who sees the world as the great champions of human freedom do—Friedrich Nietzsche, Martin Heidegger, and Jean-Paul Sartre, among others—somehow convinced Peter that how he feels and what he does have something to do with how he uses *his* freedom to construct his world, however he may have been limited in doing so by snags in his early development?

And then Peter produced these two sentences: "I don't see how I will ever have it [more out of life]. I don't accept that." This admission of a despised and rejected paralysis recalls the last words in Samuel Beckett's novel *The Unnamable*, "I can't go on, I'll go on." Peter the metaphysician: he *can't* do it, but he *will* do it. Is this not a statement of the fundamental human paradox, the starting point of so many of the more difficult and worthwhile things that people do?

During our twenty-third meeting, Peter spontaneously issued this declaration: "There has been a definite improvement in how I'm feeling and sleeping. I'm almost back to where I was before this happened." Granting this, Peter feels that he is currently at what he calls a "standstill." After 5 months, the acute anxiety he felt, along with the portent of his annihilation, is gone. But he is still stuck with the person he has been all his life, and he no longer wants to be that person.

Wondering out loud how this had all happened to him, he talked for the first time in our meetings about his childhood and his mother—it took 5 months for him to get around to talking about this woman. She was a Russian Jewish immigrant who spoke only fair English. She did not have an active social life. Peter had playmates but he was not particularly popular. He was not very coordinated and "hated" physical education. "I never felt confident about anything from the earliest age," he told me. When he was in the first grade, he wondered if he could put his belt on right.

I asked Peter how he dealt with these feelings of inferiority. "I had a smart mouth. I still can't stop doing this now. I do it over and over. If I didn't do that, I'd be a mute. If you have confidence, you don't need to do this. I can't bring myself to talk to others in a positive way. It feels phony when I do this."

At our twenty-fourth meeting, these next words came spontaneously from Peter, seeming to originate from some place deep inside him. "It's not the situation. It's the mental uncomfortableness I feel with it. None of these situations [the issues and problems that come up repeatedly during our meetings] were as bad as I thought at first." After hearing this, I asked myself if reality had finally broken through the faulty cognitive and emotional structures that had constituted Peter's neurotic world for so long.

Then came this nugget of wisdom: "You really have to hurt before you can begin to change." Peter has often complained about the pain he has had to endure as a result of the work we are doing. Now he seems to be saying that it was necessary to suffer to get to where he is, and that it was worth it. Then Peter said, "It isn't an impossible task." He has often remarked how "hard" this was going to be. His emphasis seems to have shifted from the *difficulty* of crawling out of his cocoon to the *possibility* and the *likelihood* of his being able to make this transition. I pointed out that these changes in his thinking meant real progress toward his goal of living a less anxious and restricted life. Almost reluctantly, reflecting his basic negativism and conservatism, Peter agreed with me.

Consolidation With Gradual Improvement (16 Months, 59 Meetings)

At some point—it is not clear just when—I was able to convince Peter's psychiatrist that Peter did not have a primary mood disorder and that his diagnosis of bipolar II was not right. Shortly after that, the Tegretol taper was started. By the time we met for the twenty-sixth time, Peter was off Tegretol and on a maintenance dose of BuSpar. He felt this drug was helping him to cope better and that it was not causing him any problems. He continued to believe that Tegretol had done him no good and sometimes made him dizzy.

"I don't like the idea that I can't function well without BuSpar," Peter told me, as he extolled the virtues of this drug. Clearly, he is one of those patients who do not want to depend too much on medication, though he seemed willing to let BuSpar be his pharmacological crutch for a while. Peter is feeling better, looking better, and looking ahead to a time when he will have changed enough to no longer need any medication. He told me how he had recently overcome several inclinations to go with his habitual negative thinking and how doing this changed a likely bad outcome into a relatively good one. "I want to change people's perception of me. I want to change my own self-perception," he said with conviction.

Peter made it clear that his relationship with his mother had been fraught with conflict. "Screaming and yelling" were a large part of their dialogue. He claimed that he "never resolved anything with her." He had nursed both of his parents to their deaths—his father for 2 years, and later, his mother for 6 years. Several days before his mother died, she refused the food her son was trying to spoon into her mouth. Peter, losing his temper, forced the spoon, slightly cutting the inside of her mouth. "I can't forgive myself for what I did," he said of this incident. On the morning she died, her last words to him were "Go to hell."

Though Peter did not talk much about his mother (and not at all about his father), I feel I can safely infer that, with a nod to Donald Winnicott, this woman was a "bad-enough" mother for her son to have had a neurotic development which, unredeemed, led to his neurotic adult life. Most likely, the acid of the family conflict ate into Peter's psyche, keeping him from making a solid attachment to the world that was unfolding around him as he grew. At the same time, this tenuous attachment to others and the world was, no doubt, imprinted on brain centers that underlie emotion, turning his "emotional idle" up into the range of high anxiety (this is epigenetic imprinting, and not, as Peter believed, genetic inheritance). A pathological life at the level of neurosis was his fate—he had no borderline or psychotic traits—culminating in the episode of the 5 days of emotional free fall that brought him into therapy.

At our twenty-eighth meeting, as Peter read from a list of concerns he had voiced many times before, I listened for the subtext of his words and took note of his affect. His voice was steadier than I had ever heard it before. His face had a glow, and the frown that had been so prominent before was all but gone. Peter's words told me he was still engaging the issues that he came to therapy with. His body language said things were going better for him.

During our next three meetings, Peter continued to delve into the reasons for his angry outbursts. "I feel like being angry as the first response is me—anything else is phony," he told me. He readily acknowledged that this kind of retaliation often brings on a counter-retaliation by the object of his anger, which then leads Peter into another cycle of worry and paranoia. He sees this kind of response as a part of what he calls his "internal need." Where does this "need" come from? Peter eventually acknowledged that his mother reacted to anything that displeased her with anger (though this distemper dissipated rather quickly), and that she was angry at him most of the time. It seems that Peter learned anger at his mother's knee—then kept on being angry at everyone else he met because he did not know anything else.

Peter's weakened Ego cannot live comfortably with the ambiguity that arises when, as so often happens, someone fails to live up to his expectations. Then Peter attacks what he takes to be another person's "phoniness" with the anti-phoniness club of his anger. With his angry transformation of the event's meaning, he tries to break through the moral ambiguity of these distressing situations by reasserting his challenged sense of self, in the doomed hope of making things the way they *should* be. Using this maneuver, Peter can momentarily reshape the world through his anger, defensively dealing with emotions that he cannot deal with without this defense. He knows that most people do not need the defenses he uses. He wants to join their ranks.

I asked Peter what he feels as he goes off on one of his angry transformations: "You SOB. This is the way I feel. If you don't like it, too bad." Then he added: "Why do I have to go into it like that? Why do I get so upset? I would like to think about it in a different way. Is it neurotic to think this way?" Peter feels personally wounded when someone does not meet his standards. He spoke of the "intense need to get back at the person verbally." While doing his volunteer work at the library, a woman lawyer told him that she should not have to pay a fine because she does not finish work until after the library closes, and could not have brought the books back on time. "You want something for nothing," was Peter's response. In Peter's world, the woman is still responsible for paying the fine. Later, he felt ashamed about how he had snapped at her and wished he had said something like, "These are the rules."

One of Peter's recurring themes has been the headaches that have plagued him for years and which wax and wane with his stress level, his allergies, and the medication he takes. Unlike some patients who have varying degrees of belief in the magical power of prescribed drugs, Peter implicitly believes—as I do—that the solution to the array of problems we have been chipping away at for the last 8 months depends on his will to overcome the structural deficits of a neurotic development. He does not want any improvement he has already made, or will make, to come from some pill, because that would seem false. (Put another way, he does not want to "listen to BuSpar" to feel "better than well," as Peter Kramer's patients "listen to Prozac.") Peter has spoken with his psychiatrist about reducing his dosage of BuSpar, and the tapering has begun. He wants to see if he can maintain his current degree of emotional control while taking less of the drug. I see this as a move to take more control of his healing process, and as a very positive sign.

By our thirty-sixth meeting, Peter had discontinued BuSpar. A week later, he reported no difference in his anxiety level or mood. But the headaches persisted, a dull pain that hit him most when he was not doing anything. Though Peter has put more activity in his life, mostly through his volunteer work, he still has periods of empty time when he feels dragged down by boredom. Shortly after stopping BuSpar, he had his last meeting with his psychiatrist. By that time, all three of us were convinced that medication was not going to fix Peter. Though their parting was amicable, Peter gave no indication of regretting the loss of either his psychiatrist or the drugs he had prescribed. Nor did he appear angry about the misdiagnosis that was made—I was candid with him about this. The forgiveness and generosity Peter showed here surprised me. As is obvious from most of what he says, his stance toward the rest of the world was anything but forgiving and generous.

The way I see things now, Peter is continuing to do therapeutic work on a gradually rising plateau. He still struggles with many of the issues he came in with, but in a more existential and less neurotic way. He is internalizing the lessons learned during our meetings, and growing from this experience. What keeps him moving forward, I believe, is that his life on the plateau does not give him the satisfaction he craves. The inertia of his faulty development holds him back, even as he tries to move forward: "I still can't see myself doing certain things. I'm afraid to get into something because of the headaches and flushing that might come." Peter continues to fight anticipatory anxiety. And, he told me again for the hundredth time, the negative thoughts are still with him.

The final sentence of my chart note for our thirty-ninth meeting read: "Peter looks better now than at any time since we started nine months ago." I felt that some milestone had been reached. He described the preceding week as "fair, better," and his headaches were down. "Are my worries subsiding or did the headaches become less because I stopped using Becanase?" he asked. [This was a drug he was taking for a stuffy nose.] "I would like to get to the point where, if I have something I can't resolve, I won't worry to excess, and get a headache or a hot flash." Some of Peter's current worries are: his next-door neighbor is planning to move and he is concerned about who will buy the house; he is having some repair work done on his own house and he wonders if the work will be done right and if he will be overcharged; he is still concerned that if he does not push himself to do more, he will not improve in the way he wants to improve. Peter has gone back to his exercise program at the Jewish community center, on Monday, Wednesday, and Friday. Mostly, he uses the treadmill.

On his gradually rising plateau, Peter is trying to balance his need to do more with the need not to be overwhelmed by worry and anxiety as he takes on new projects. He points with pride to the small jobs he does around his house and yard. He recently planted 36 small annual plants in his back yard and fixed an aluminum awning. This is in contrast to the paralysis he felt a year ago when he was heading into the crisis that brought him to therapy. "Last year, I didn't get anything accomplished," he told me. "In the back of my mind, I'm still scared that things will slide back, although things are going well." Peter has not complained recently about disturbed sleep, and his outbursts, which have been such a big problem all his life, were not even mentioned today.

"The thoughts go through my mind … a semi-boring life … I wonder if I might slip back to what got me here in the first place … no job … not ready to date … discouraging … this is the rest of my life … boring … not fulfilling … there's more to me than this boring life." As I listened to Peter's stream of consciousness about life on his plateau, with all its limitations and frustrations, I believe I heard something closer to an existential cry from the depths than the neurotic productions I had become accustomed to hearing. When I made this interpretation, he appeared to understand.

During our forty-third meeting, 10 months after we started, Peter announced that two more months might be the right amount of time to continue our work. Frankly, I was stunned that he was even considering terminating at this point. Some "remaining issues," he said, needed to be discussed. One of these issues was his sexuality, or, as he put it, the lack of his sexuality. "I am as close to being a virgin as a man can be," he told me. It was obvious from the beginning that Peter had a deeply seated fear of getting involved with a woman. The very *idea* paralyzes him, even now.

When he used the words "fear of homosexuality," I asked him to explain what he was afraid of. "My loneliness … Could something happen between a man I like … I don't think I could have a physical relationship with a man … Kiss a man … Have anal sex … I don't think I could handle it." He mentioned a man he knew when he was in the Air Force. The man was homosexual and they became friends. One day, he asked Peter to rub his back. Peter saw this as a sexual overture and declined. He wanted me to understand that he had "no desire" to start a sexual relationship with this man. My initial reaction was that being so sexually inexperienced, Peter could not totally reject the notion that a man might provide for him what he was never bold enough to ask a woman for.

At several of our earlier meetings, Peter talked about the problem he had concentrating on any written text or film that has intellectual or emotional substance. "I'm afraid to look at it, afraid to get into it," he told me during our forty-fifth meeting. Whether it is the real world or the world of fiction, issues involving emotional conflict seem to send out a "stop" signal that paralyzes him. As part of my ongoing effort to prod Peter up the grade of his plateau, I recommended that he select a book or film of the type he has trouble with, take it on, and let the chips fall where they may. He had previously tried to watch a video of *The Shawshank Redemption*, a movie set mostly in a prison, with a stunning performance and voice-over by Morgan Freeman. He could not see it to the end. He agreed to try again. The next week the report was good: "I liked it. It felt like a triumph that I did it. Got over the hump on it." Peter gave a vivid, detailed, and animated account of the story. He enjoyed sharing this victory with me, adding, "Like a lot of things in my life, I wouldn't do something if someone didn't push me to do it." He acknowledged me as his "pusher" on this project. Peter's watching this movie entailed the clearing of a blockage—the same kind of blockage, no doubt, that had kept him from going for so many things all his life. "I can't figure out why I do this," he said with what appeared to be genuine wonder. Earlier, Peter had admitted to "tuning out" what others were saying during one-to-one conversations. He has, in fact, tuned out large segments of the world, a practice that has left him isolated and unfulfilled. We have been uncovering the meanings of his refusal of the world and are challenging the psychological structures that underlie and drive it.

For all of Peter's complaining about how non-ideal life on his plateau is, he has, during the last few months, put together a productive daily schedule. Peter clocks 20 hours a week as a volunteer with senior citizens at the Jewish community center; he gives two hours a week as a volunteer in the pulmonary unit at a local hospital; and he volunteers another two hours at a library near his home. He appears to be doing well in this work. It is when Peter is not at one of these venues that time rests heavily on him, that he becomes bored and worried and gets down on himself. He does not enjoy doing anything alone, but is too conflicted about the intentions of others to consistently seek out compatible company. "It's depressing going out by myself," he told me. "Everyone else is with someone else."

At our fifty-first meeting, just one year after we began, Peter told me he had come to feel that the medication he had been taking may have done him more harm than good. "I don't think I'm the kind of person medicine works on," he said. "I took the medicine because I was so desperate." He recently stopped Seldane for his allergies. The headaches that had plagued him for so long disappeared. As a somaticizer and a hypochondriac, hoping to find relief from various symptoms, Peter has taken a good deal of medicine. He has a low threshold for physical pain, as well as emotional pain. That Peter is now willing to let go of his pharmacological crutches seems a big step forward. As he discontinues one drug after another, including his psychotropic drugs, he gives no indication of wanting to go back on any of them. Three weeks after stopping Seldane, he has yet to have another significant headache. "It's like night and day," he said.

Two weeks later, Peter gave this progress report. "What the hell am I going to whine about today? I'm on a plateau [he's picked up my metaphor], which isn't so bad. Some time has to pass before anything more happens, before I can do anything better … At the back of my mind I think things are not so bad but could be better. I think about the ideal. I would meet a woman and … but I don't think about the negative [way things could go]. Maybe right now I'm not ready for this. I'm feeling good now. I don't have many down, negative days now. I guess the right thing is to plunge right in, but I might not be ready. If I think about it, I can get discouraged. If I cope day to day, something good will happen. That's where I am now."

These are Peter's most hopeful words yet. Life is not all he would hope it to be, but he is coping with his situation now and looking ahead, if tentatively, to a time when he will have more of what he wants. And he seems to be willing to work for it.

"I'm almost back to where I was a year ago," Peter let it be known during our next meeting. "But there is a difference. I have a better understanding of how I deal with people. I feel better about a lot of things. But I'm on that plateau. I think of that as a little depressing. I keep plugging, day by day. I can only work on things I am working on now." Peter had only one headache last week, which was quickly resolved with an over-the-counter pain medication. He attributes his improved sleep to the absence of the headaches that have bothered him for so long.

The next month and a half was mostly taken up with a wider and deeper exploration of the joys and sorrows of Peter's life on the plateau. He recently took a bus trip to Atlantic City with a friend. The day went well, and he appeared pleased. This does not seem like much of an accomplishment until it is recalled that, one year earlier, he attempted a similar excursion, but was too anxious to even get on the bus. The uneasiness Peter is feeling now, and discusses at length at every meeting, is a prerequisite for his continuing growth. His dilemma hurts him more on some days than on others. Peter is learning to raise the threshold of his emotional pain. He realizes that he cannot get to where he wants to go until this low tolerance is overcome.

This is not easy. The incidents Peter has discussed at our meetings that have caused him pain all have the same form. Some encounter with another person results in his becoming anxious (at a low threshold); Peter then fears that his anxiety will increase and that the dreaded somatic symptoms (headache, flushing, disturbed sleep) will reappear; his anxiety increases; he aborts the encounter in hope of discharging the anxiety; he feels regret and frustration at defaulting on the situation. A day or so later, he lets go of these negative feelings, acknowledging to himself and to me that there was never anything to really be anxious about.

Clearly, Peter never learned the art of self-soothing. Most people facing the situations that overwhelm him are able to talk themselves down from the initial anxious feelings that often come with new challenges. Peter cannot do this. Instead, he replays in his head what cognitive therapists call "old tapes" of bad experiences. This projected negativity sends his anxiety into high gear and through the cognitive-behavioral loop just sketched. Peter implicitly understands this: "This is the way I'm used to doing things, the way I learned to function." From what Peter has told me about his mother, it is not hard to see why.

The following words were spoken by Peter at our sixty-sixth meeting: "I'm afraid to believe that I don't let things get me down now as much as I used to. I seem to be better. I don't want to believe it. Nothing positive like that can happen in my life. I'm coping better." If I hear him correctly, Peter is telling me that he fears *not* being as negativistic as he has always been! Even if it is painful, his negative, neurotic life is predictable—he can count on the same anxious pain and on his identity as the one who is experiencing that pain. But what would a less negativistic life be like for him? What new demands would the world make then? I told Peter that expressing his fear about the improvement he sees in himself is good evidence that he is improving. Peter's next task is to find something positive to replace his negative life with.

The ups and downs of Peter's life continued to be reported and discussed at the meetings that followed. Then, at our seventieth meeting, came this declaration: "It seems I have gone as far as I can go with therapy. I'm not really making progress the way I want to make it." Despite the fact that Peter continued to struggle with what seemed to be the same issues, it is clear to me that he was struggling more effectively and at a higher level. Acknowledgments such as "Before I started coming here, I did not understand what was going on with me," made with conviction and a sense of gratitude, convinced me that our work was having its intended effect. When I asked what the next step should be, he responded, "I can't imagine giving up coming here." I suggested that we meet every other week, instead of weekly, as we have been doing. Peter rejected the idea, saying that he still needs the "support" he gets from our sessions and appreciates the opportunity to "ventilate" his feelings. Though Peter is frustrated with the "stuck" aspect of life on his plateau, he is seeing some forward movement there as well. He still works hard at our meetings. He is not just "feeding," as the psychoanalysts describe the situation where patients come in mostly to have their infantile needs met.

Peter came to our seventy-forth meeting with this extraordinary revelation, which made it easier to understand why his life had been a living death: "I can't stand the anxiety of waiting for the situation to be over. I want all worry taken out of my mind." What Peter is ultimately saying here is that he does not want any ambiguity, uncertainty, or risk in his life.

I pointed out that he was, in effect, *demanding* that the world not be an ambiguous, uncertain place, where risks must be taken. Put another way, Peter had refused to take life on life's terms. He wanted his own terms! He wanted a "privileged" life where he does not have to play by the same rules as everyone else.

The good news is that Peter is not refusing life on life's terms as doggedly as he had done for most of his life. The following declaration, made during our seventy-fifth meeting, shows that Peter has come a long way in challenging the psychological structures that have made his life so problematic: "Anything that would really bother me before I am tolerating it better now." At the next meeting, he said: "I am 100% better than I was two years ago." Clearly, he is not 100% better, but he is slowly making it up his plateau.

"I want perfection," Peter told me at our seventy-seventh meeting. "I guess that's why I like fantasy stories [and initially why he had trouble watching *The Shawshank Redemption*] … I've always had the expectation that friendships would be forever, perfect … a certain level of neuroticism … I can't completely overcome it … I have to accept life more like it is." These words gave me hope that Peter had internalized the interpretation I made three weeks earlier, as I pointed out why he wants all imperfection removed from his life, so he can have the "perfect" life. He seems to understand that, in making this claim on the world, he is asking for more trouble of the kind he has always had.

Our seventy-ninth meeting was our last weekly meeting. A month later, Peter came up with these words that both recalled where we had been and adumbrated where he still hoped to go: "I've been thinking that I won't be coming here any more. Seems like the right time to end. Whatever I haven't resolved that I would like to resolve … I've done the best I can … I would like to accomplish more, but … I may have had an unrealistic idea that I could just go out there and date and be comfortable … I don't think I'll be able to push that any further than I have … Sometimes you just can't have all the things you want … Now I won't have anyone to talk to, I'll just have to do it on my own." Here was a powerful account of a painful resolution of what had been an agonizing conflict.

Peter had made the decision to end our work at this time. He looked well and seemed in control. I saw little of the agony that was so evident during the last 20 months. I felt Peter had learned enough to be his own therapist now—to keep pushing up the grade of his plateau. How much had Peter improved? I would say he was 30–40% better when he walked out the door for the last time than when he first came through it.

We met once more, a month later. "I now have a doubt … Maybe I could understand this better … Am I just trying to prolong my therapy because

I don't want to quit? … Why can't I be the kind of person who doesn't get upset when things aren't the way I feel they should be? … Perhaps it's that I don't have a wife to go home to … grandchildren." This seemed like the kind of doubt and questioning that would keep Peter honest and moving forward. Looking back, I could only wonder where he had found the ego strength to do the work we did.

I told Peter that, if he wanted to meet again, the door was always open. He never walked through it again. During the years since we finished our work, he has called several times to say he was doing well, continuing with his volunteer work, going places with friends, and, yes, becoming involved with a woman or two. I saw him at performances of the local symphony orchestra, usually accompanied by another person. Peter looked good, sounded good, and appeared pleased that we had run into each other. It seems that the grade of the plateau he reached when we were meeting kept rising.

Notes

Chapter 1: Seeing Through the Illusion of Biological Psychiatry

1. René J. Muller, *Psych ER: Psychiatric Patients Come to the Emergency Room* (Hillsdale, NJ: The Analytic Press, 2003).
2. The current standard of practice in diagnosing a mental disorder is that patients must meet the behavioral criteria established for the disorder by the *Diagnostic and Statistical Manual of Mental Disorders*, 4th ed. (*DSM-IV*) (Washington, DC: American Psychiatric Association, 1994).
3. Conrad M. Swartz, "Antipsychotic Psychosis," *Psychiatric Times* (October 2004): 17–20. Examples with literature citations are given here of patients who developed psychotic symptoms either after using antipsychotic medication for an extended period or after suddenly stopping these drugs, precipitating a "discontinuation syndrome" that is thought to be brought on by dopaminergic hypersensitivity. See also Peter R. Breggin, *Toxic Psychiatry: Why Therapy, Empathy, and Love Must Replace the Drugs, Electroshock, and Biochemical Theories of the "New Psychiatry"* (New York: St. Martin's Press, 1991), pp. 85–86.
4. Neuroleptic and atypical antipsychotic drugs, some more than others, have been shown to extend the electrocardiographic QT_c interval in certain patients. This interval is a measure of the time it takes for the heart muscle to repolarize after a contraction. QT_c prolongation has been associated with a particularly nasty arrythmia that can lead to sudden death. For a general discussion of this phenomenon see Barbara A. Liu and David N. Juurlink, "Drugs and the QT Interval—Caveat Doctor," *New England Journal of Medicine* 351 (2004): 1053–1056. For a perspective on psychotropic drugs and QT_c prolongation see Michael J. Labellarte, "Assessing Risk of QT_c Prolongation," *Psychiatric Times* (May 2004): 49–53. Neuroleptics and atypical antipsychotic medications, as well as some mood stabilizers, are known to cause weight gain and hyperglycemia; see Hua Jin and Jonathan M. Meyer, "Glucose Dysregulation," *Psychiatric Times* (March 2003): 22–24.

5. Peter D. Kramer, *Listening to Prozac: A Psychiatrist Explores Antidepressant Drugs and the Remaking of the Self* (New York: Penguin Books, 1994), p. x. Kramer's book became a publishing phenomenon. The "wow" response of some who took Prozac encouraged both patients and clinicians to believe that depression really was caused by a "chemical imbalance," and that Prozac had corrected it. Not everyone who took this drug and felt "better than well" realized that others who had earlier taken prescription doses of amphetamine and cocaine had a similar response to these drugs (Joseph Glenmullen, *Prozac Backlash: Overcoming the Dangers of Prozac, Zoloft, Paxil, and Other Antidepressants with Safe, Effective Alternatives* [New York: Simon & Schuster, 2000], pp. 214–217); see also Joseph Glenmullen, *The Antidepressant Solution: A Step-by-Step Guide to Safely Overcoming Antidepressant Withdrawal, Dependence, and "Addiction"* (New York: Free Press, 2005).
6. Psychiatrists, psychologists, and philosophers who have the existential perspective on the world in general and on mental illness in particular posit the notion of the authentic self, a condition of Being that can never be fully achieved, but only approached. Herbert Fingarette wrote a brief, incisive book on self-deception, which is one way we have of acting inauthentically (*Self-Deception* [Atlantic Highlands, NJ: Humanities Press, 1969]). Self-deception is a major theme in my first book, *The Marginal Self: An Existential Inquiry Into Narcissism* (Atlantic Highlands, NJ: Humanities Press International, 1987), and its sequel, *Beyond Marginality: Constructing a Self in the Twilight of Western Culture* (Westport, CT: Praeger, 1998).
7. "It is not enough to say that we live in a world where betrayal is possible at every moment and in every form: betrayal of all by all and of each by himself. I repeat, this betrayal seems pressed upon us by the very shape of our world" (Gabriel Marcel, *Being and Having: An Existentialist Diary*, Trans. Katherine Farrer [New York: Harper Torchbooks, 1965], p. 97).
8. Charles Mackay, *Extraordinary Popular Delusions & the Madness of Crowds*, with a Foreword by Andrew Tobias (New York: Three Rivers Press, 1841/1980).
9. Quoted by Alan Stone in *Psychiatric Times* (April 2004): 16.
10. I do not mean to imply here that artists are emotionally healthy because of their insight, or that they routinely heal themselves or others through their art. Knowing what a healthy response would be does not guarantee one will make that response.
11. Albert Camus, "The Artist as Witness of Freedom: The Independent Mind in an Age of Ideologies," *Commentary* (December 1949): 543–538. "By his very function, the artist is the witness of freedom, and this is a justification for which he sometimes pays dearly. By his function he is engaged in the density of history, where man's very flesh stifles."

Chapter 2: How Biological Psychiatry Lost the Mind and Went Brain Dead

1. Alix Spiegel, "The Dictionary of Disorder: How One Man Revolutionized Psychiatry," *New Yorker*, January 3, 2005, 56–63.

2. Nancy C. Andreasen, *Brave New Brain: Conquering Mental Illness in the Era of the Genome* (New York: Oxford University Press, 2001).
3. Thomas H. Lee and Lee Goldman, "Evaluation of the Patient with Acute Chest Pain," *New England Journal of Medicine* 342 (2000): 1187–1195.
4. Paul Genova, "Dump the *DSM*!" *Psychiatric Times* (April 2003): 72–75.
5. Nutan A. Vaidya and Michael A. Taylor, "The *DSM*: Should It Have a Future?" *Psychiatric Times* (March 2006): 73–79.
6. Andreasen, *Brave New Brain*, p. 183.
7. René J. Muller, "An ER Patient with a Personality Disorder Misdiagnosed as Schizophrenia," *Psychiatric Times* (January 1999): 37–38; and "Comment" *Psychiatric Times* (June 1999): 73–74.
8. Ross J. Baldessarini, "A Plea for Integrity of the Bipolar Concept," *Bipolar Disorder* 2 (2000): 3–7.
9. The *DSM-IV* quotations were taken from the first and last paragraphs of the section titled "Definition of Mental Disorder," *DSM-IV*, xxi–xxii.
10. Ibid.
11. Gabriel Marcel, *Being and Having*, p. 64.
12. Nancy C. Andreasen, *The Broken Brain: The Biological Revolution in Psychiatry* (New York: Oxford University Press, 1984).
13. R.D. Laing, *The Divided Self: An Existential Study in Sanity and Madness* (Baltimore: Penguin Books, 1965).
14. The downside of biological psychiatry's transformation of mind into matter is parsed by Carl Zimmer, *Soul Made Flesh: The Discovery of the Brain and How It Changed the World* (New York: Free Press, 2004).
15. Marcia Angell, a former editor of the *New England Journal of Medicine*, faced this issue head-on in *The Truth About the Drug Companies: How They Deceive Us and What to Do About It* (New York: Random House, 2004). The drug companies have a stake in maintaining our contemporary version of the inauthentic society, which tends to favor the development of psychiatric symptoms (all social orders seem to exert a strong pathological influence). Big Pharma, backed by third-party payers for mental health and by biological psychiatry, ultimately works against challenging the reasons behind patients' symptoms in favor of smoothing these symptoms over with medication. The idea that psychiatric symptoms often are a sign that something is wrong in a person's life that needs remediation—as somatic symptoms signal a medical problem that requires treatment—is denied and covered up. The status quo of our inauthentic society is preserved because drug companies, insurers, and doctors are a part of that society and are paid to preserve it, participants as they are in a culture of greed.
16. The apt term "medicalization of discontent" was used by Meika Loe in *The Rise of Viagra: How the Little Blue Pill Changed Sex in America* (New York: New York University Press, 2004).
17. Mortimer J. Adler's *How to Read a Book: The Art of Getting a Liberal Education* (New York: Simon & Schuster, 1960) taught me a great deal about how to approach a nonfiction text. John Ciardi's *How Does a Poem Mean?* (Cambridge, MA: The Riverside Press, 1959) did the same for poetry. Two giants from the faculty of Columbia University spoke to my youthful, idealistic self: Gilbert Highet, *The Art of Teaching* (New York: Vintage Books, 1950); and Jacques Barzun, *Teacher in America* (Garden City, NY: Anchor Books, 1954).

18. Arnold Weinstein, *A Scream Goes Through the House: What Literature Teaches Us about Life* (New York: Random House, 2003), p. 73. In a similar vein, Alain de Botton saw Marcel Proust's multivolume novel *In Search of Lost Time* as a text to be mined for psychological insights—as well as being one of the twentieth century's greatest literary works. The following excerpt from his book *How Proust Can Change Your Life* (New York: Vintage Books, 1998), p. 72, is about inauthentic, or pathological, suffering: "Proust's novel is filled with those we might call *bad sufferers*, wretched souls who have been betrayed in love or excluded from parties, who are pained by a feeling of intellectual inadequacy or a sense of social inferiority, but who learn nothing from such ills, and indeed react to them by engaging in a variety of ruinous defense mechanisms which entail arrogance and delusion, cruelty and callousness, spite and rage." You can just *feel* neurotic defenses being played out here, even without knowing the characters or the story. By showing how the bad choices these characters made disfigured their lives and the lives of others, we might be encouraged to find more authentic and healthful ways of responding the next time we find ourselves betrayed by the world.

    Abraham Verghese has written about how his experience with literature has helped him to become a better physician: "good literature, particularly fiction, has the power to transform"; "A well-developed fiction-reading capacity allows us to imagine our patients' worlds fully and put ourselves in their shoes" ("The Calling," *New England Journal of Medicine* 352 [2005]: 1844–1847). In a review of Ian McEwan's novel *Saturday* (New York: Talese/Doubleday, 2005), Zoe Heller notes: "[L]iterature cannot give absolute answers, or furnish watertight explanations. What it can do, McEwan proposes, is capture the moral tangle of personal life and historical context that is our lived experience" *(The New York Times Book Review*, March 20, 2005, 1, 10, 11).

    Dinko Podrug has used Shakespeare's *Hamlet* as a model to teach psychiatric residents about pursuing patients' stories to uncover their authentic meaning. "Watching Hamlet, I was struck with how this play's action is, like that of no other, propelled by the main characters' systematic efforts to find out—to extract from one another—the hidden truth" ("Through *Hamlet* to Narrative Medicine and Neuroscience: Literature as a Basic Science of Psychiatry," *Psychiatric Times* (June 2005): 23–25).
19. *The William Carlos Williams Reader*, edited and with an introduction by M.L. Rosenthal (New York: New Directions, 1966), pp. 73–74. The excerpt quoted here comes at the end of this long poem, which dates from 1955.
20. Heller, 1, 10, 11.
21. Quoted in John Leland, "It's Only Rhyming Quatrains, But I Like It," *The New York Times Magazine*, July 8, 2001, 36–39.
22. Someone who grasps that self-deception is a universal phenomenon—that we often lie to ourselves about many things—might be expected to spot a specific instance of self-deception, such as the one being vetted here. If psychiatrists were better schooled in existential philosophy, would they be less self-deceived? This outcome is by no means certain: a good deal of history (as well as my own personal experience) is not reassuring. The capacity to identify an authentic response does not guarantee one will make that response.

23. Upton Sinclair (1878–1968) was a crusading—some say "muckraking"—journalist whose best-known work was the *The Jungle*, a novel about the abuses of the meatpacking industry in the early twentieth century. The citation here is taken from Paul Krugman, "Harvest of Lemons," *The New York Times*, October 10, 2001, 13.
24. Rollo May, *The Courage to Create* (New York: W.W. Norton, 1975), pp. 124–125.

Chapter 3: The Brain Cannot Account for What We Think, Feel, and Do

1. Kramer, *Listening to Prozac*, p. 297.
2. Jean-Paul Sartre, *Nausea, The Wall and Other Stories*, Trans. Lloyd Alexander; introduction Hayden Carruth (New York: MJF Books, 1964), pp. 99–100. Sartre uses the word *nothingness* here to signify the inauthentic refusal of life, a kind of non-being, the way Roquentin lived before his epiphany of authentic existence. In *Being and Nothingness*, Sartre uses this word to mean something entirely different: *Nothingness*—no-thing-ness—specifies a state of human being that is marked by consciousness and freedom, which is never fully itself and always in formation—that is, not a thing. *Being*, on the other hand, specifies the existence of an inanimate, thing-like being without consciousness or freedom (a cow, a tree, a table), which has its essence given to it once and for all, cannot change itself, and can only be altered by some external force (unlike a person, who must create his existence moment to moment). These terms, paradoxical as they may seem, are basic to Sartre's ontology (Jean-Paul Sartre, *Being and Nothingness: An Essay on Phenomenological Ontology*, Trans. and with an introduction by Hazel E. Barnes [New York: Philosophical Library, 1956]).
3. And another reminder of how right Gabriel Marcel was when he wrote that "we live in a world where betrayal is possible at every moment ..." (*Being and Having*, p. 97).
4. See Robert M. Pirsig, *Zen and the Art of Motorcycle Maintenance* (New York: Bantam Books, 1974). Pirsig's novel shows how the Cartesian take on life can incline some individuals toward psychopathology, and conversely how existential thought, correctly understood and lived, can heal. I owe a great debt to that broad spectrum of thinkers and writers who are collectively known for their "existential" take on the world. Many books could be cited in explication of this tradition. I will offer these: William Barrett, *Irrational Man: A Study in Existential Philosophy* (New York: Anchor Books, 1962); Ralph Harper, *The Existential Experience* (Baltimore: The Johns Hopkins University Press, 1972); Muller, *The Marginal Self* and the sequel, *Beyond Marginality*. The philosophical anthropology underlying these texts is a touchstone for the critique of psychiatry I am making here.
5. Francis Crick, *The Astonishing Hypothesis: The Scientific Search for the Soul* (New York: Touchstone, 1994), p. 3. See Mark Steyn, "The Twentieth-Century Darwin: Francis Crick (1916–2004)," *Atlantic Monthly*, October 2004, 206–207. "But just as a joke that's explained is no longer funny, so in his final Astonishing Hypothesis, Dr. Crick eventually arrived at the logical end: you can unmask the mystery of humanity only by denying our humanity."

6. Andreasen, *Brave New Brain*, p. 41. The following books spell out the hit psychiatric patients took when what was formerly credited to the mind was appropriated for the brain. Robert Whitaker, *Mad in America: Bad Science, Bad Medicine, and the Enduring Mistreatment of the Mentally Ill* (Cambridge, MA: Perseus Publishing, 2002); and Peter Zachar, *Psychological Concepts and Biological Psychiatry: A Philosophical Analysis. Advances in Philosophical Analysis*, Vol. 28 (Philadelphia: John Benjamins Publishing Co., 2000).
7. For a discussion of brain diseases that produce psychiatric sequelae see D. Frank Benson and Dietrich Blumer, Eds., *Psychiatric Aspects of Neurologic Disease*, Vol. 2 (New York: Grune & Stratton, 1982).
8. Andreasen, *Brave New Brain*, p. 113.
9. Ibid., p. 127. Schizophrenia remains the most illusive of the mental illnesses. The borna virus was once thought to infect only horses and sheep. But when antibodies to the virus were found in the blood of some schizophrenic patients, researchers began looking for evidence that the virus played a causative role. Commenting on the data from one study, William T. Carpenter, Jr., director of the Maryland Psychiatric Research Center, noted, "There are very few leads in schizophrenia research" (Kristy Wooley, "Rare Virus May Be Linked to Schizophrenia," *Albion Monitor*, December 3, 1995, www.monitor.net/monitor). A leading schizophrenia researcher acknowledges here that no one has much of an idea about what causes this mental disorder. The fact that the borna virus has attracted serious attention as a possible culprit could be taken to mean that, in the absence of any solid evidence, scientists are not above clutching at straws.
10. Andreasen, *Brave New Brain*, p. 41.
11. Ibid, p. 341.
12. Ibid.
13. Ibid, p. 342.
14. *DSM-IV*, xxi.
15. Rainer Maria Rilke, *Letters to a Young Poet*, Trans. and with a foreword by Stephen Mitchell (New York: Random House, 1984), pp. 34–35. These Zen-like words encourage us to engage with the world. It seems odd that Marcel Proust, who wrote in *Remembrance of Things Past* that "the only true paradise is always the paradise we have lost," would also issue this warning against taking what is written about the world for the world itself: "Reading becomes dangerous when instead of waking us to the personal life of the spirit, it tends to substitute itself for it, when truth no longer appears to us as an ideal we can realize only through the intimate progress of our thought and the effort of our heart, but as a material thing, deposited between the leaves of books like honey ready-made by others, and which we have only to take the trouble of reaching for on the shelves of libraries and then savoring passively in perfect repose of body and mind." Quoted in Anthony Lane, "Beyond a Joke: The Perils of Loving P.G. Wodehouse," *New Yorker*, April 19 & 26, 2004, 138–149. Proust would not be the first writer to warn others against what he himself could not avoid doing. Sartre's Roquentin succumbed to this same self-loss-through-writing trap before having his "I exist …" epiphany.

Chapter 4: The Lost Art of Psychiatric Diagnosis

1. *Stedman's Medical Dictionary*, 26th ed. (Baltimore: Williams & Wilkins, 1995), p. 736.
2. *DSM-IV*, xvii–xviii.
3. The following articles go a long way toward pointing out the weaknesses of the *DSM*: Genova, "Dump the *DSM*!" (a counterpoint argument is offered by Michael First and Robert L. Spitzer: "The *DSM*: Not Perfect, but Better Than the Alternative," *Psychiatric Times* (April 2003): 73–78); Phillip M. Sinaikin, "How I Learned to Stop Worrying and Love the *DSM*," *Psychiatric Times* (February 2004): 103–105. A 1992 summary of the thoughts of Paul R. McHugh about an alternative approach to psychiatric diagnosis can be found at www.hopkinsmedicine.org/jhhpsychiatry/perspec1.htm.
4. *Phenomenology* is a word with many meanings. G. Lanteri-Laura's Chapter 4, "Phenomenology and a Critique of the Foundations of Psychiatry," in A.J.J. de Koning and F.A. Jenner, Eds., *Phenomenology and Psychiatry* (London, Academic Press, 1982), pp. 51–62, provides various definitions of this often mystifying term and shows how existential phenomenology has been used by some European psychiatrists to overcome the reductive limitations of a psychiatry dominated by biology. G.E. Berrios is less enthusiastic about the salutary effect of existential phenomenology on psychiatry: "Phenomenology and Psychopathology: Was There Ever a Relationship?" *Comprehensive Psychiatry* 34 (1993): 213–220.
5. "The Dictionary of Disorder: How One Man Revolutionized Psychiatry," *New Yorker*, January 3, 2005, 56–63. See also Mitchell Wilson, "DSM-III and the Transformation of American Psychiatry: A History," *American Journal of Psychiatry* 150 (1993): 399–410.
6. "One expression of the complex relationship between personality and affective disorder is the comorbidity of personality disorders (PDs) with affective disorders. In a sample of 117 patients with unipolar and 60 with bipolar affective disorders, we assessed DSM-III-R PDs with the Structured Clinical Interview for DSM-IV Personality Disorders (SCID-II) and compared them with personality factors as obtained by the five-factor model (FFM-NEO Five-Factor Inventory). Fifty-one percent of the unipolar and 38% of the bipolar disorders fulfilled criteria for a comorbid PD." These are the opening lines of a publication by Peter Brieger, Uwe Ehrt, and Andreas Marneros, "Frequency of Comorbid Personality Disorders in Bipolar and Unipolar Affective Disorders," *Comprehensive Psychiatry* 44 (2003): 28–34. It seems to me that the language used here immediately announces the vacuity of the comorbidity approach to understanding mental illness. Disembodied, meaningless symptoms gleaned from the SCID-II are compared with personality factors from the FFM-NEO Five-Factor Inventory. After all this abstraction and statistical manipulation, who could possibly know what is going on with any of the hapless patients who agreed to participate in this study? Comorbidity surely has a headstone in the graveyard of psychiatric misdiagnosis.
7. Martin Heidegger, *Being and Time*, Trans. John Macquarrie and Edward Robinson (New York: Harper & Row, 1962).

8. A.O. Scott, "The Hungriest Critic of Them All," *The New York Times*, June 29, Sec. 2, 1, 22.
9. This is a particular instance of the general case that realizing you do not know something can be the first step in coming to know it. A. McGhee Harvey was a professor of medicine at the Johns Hopkins University School of Medicine, and was renowned for his diagnostic skill. He taught generations of medical students using the case method of diagnosis, where the emphasis is on learning everything you can about a patient before making a diagnosis. A key element of this method is differential diagnosis: any illness that could possibly account for a patient's presentation is considered, and the less likely causes are ruled out until the most likely cause stands. Richard S. Ross, a cardiologist who trained with Harvey, described the process this way: "It's a system of lists that makes sure you think of everything. So you don't *not* make the diagnosis because you haven't thought of it" (Janet Farrar Worthington, "Portrait of a Hopkins Giant: Mac Harvey," *Hopkins Medical News* [Spring 1989]: 12–16). Ultimately a good deal of psychiatric diagnosis fails because what is really wrong with the patient is never even considered.

   According to the historian Daniel Boorstein, "The greatest obstacle to knowledge is not ignorance; it is the illusion of knowledge." Yogi Berra put it this way: "It's not what you don't know that will bite you; it's what you don't know that you don't know" (quoted by William R. Brody, "Discovery," *The [Johns Hopkins] Gazette* (November 6, 2006): 3).

Chapter 5: A Blatant Misdiagnosis of Schizophrenia

The first section of this chapter, ending with "I can only wonder where Adam might be in all this," was published earlier (René J. Muller, "Early-Morning Phone Calls From a Friend Misdiagnosed With Schizophrenia," *Psychiatric Times* (February 2002): 24–27). Major deletions were made from the middle part of the original article, and other minor changes were made throughout.

1. Muller, *The Marginal Self*, pp. 103–132.
2. R.D. Laing and D.G. Cooper, *Reason and Violence: A Decade of Sartre's Philosophy (1950–1960)* (London: Tavistock Publications, 1964), p. 7.
3. This quotation is from a secondary source, where only the name of the author, Alfred Adler, was cited. Efforts to find the original quotation were unsuccessful. A similar quotation, "Neurosis and psychosis are manifestations of discouragement," appears in *The Collected Clinical Works of Alfred Adler: Journal Articles 1921–1926*, Vol. 5 (Bellingham, WA: Alfred Adler Institute of Northwestern Washington, 2004), p. 17. Henry T. Stein, PhD helped with this identification. See also Paul Tillich, *The Courage to Be* (New Haven: Yale University Press, 1952).
4. Leslie Knowlton, "Rehabilitation: A Crucial Component of Mental Health," *Psychiatric Times* (June 2001): 13–14.
5. Erik H. Erikson, *Childhood and Society*, 2nd ed. (New York: W.W. Norton, 1963), pp. 247–251.

6. Gregory Bateson, Don D. Jackson, Jay Haley, and John Weakland, "Toward a Theory of Schizophrenia," *Behavioral Science* 1 (1956): 251–264; Gregory Bateson, Don D. Jackson, Jay Haley, and John H. Weakland, "A Note on the Double Bind—1962," *Family Process* 2 (1963): 154–161. Bateson's theory of the double bind has been important in the work of R.D. Laing (Richard I. Evans, *R.D. Laing: The Man and His Ideas* [New York: E.P. Dutton, 1976], pp. 27–28; Daniel Burston, *The Wing of Madness: The Life and Work of R.D. Laing* [Cambridge, MA: Harvard University Press, 1996]).
7. Laing, *The Divided Self.*
8. I owe the incisive turn of phrase "that which must not be known" to psychiatrist and psychoanalyst Barbara Young, MD, who proffered it while commenting on this manuscript.
9. Louis B. Fierman, Ed., *Effective Psychotherapy: The Contribution of Hellmuth Kaiser* (New York: Free Press, 1965), pp. 1–13.
10. *DSM-IV*, p. 629.
11. *Diagnostic and Statistical Manual of Mental Disorders*, 2nd ed. (*DSM-II*) (Washington, DC: American Psychiatric Association, 1968), p. 44.
12. Jerry M. Lewis, "To Hear the Cry of Bats," *Psychiatric Times* (March 2005): 43–44.

Chapter 6: How Psychiatry Created an Epidemic of Misdiagnosed Bipolar Disorder

1. Major depression "superimposed" on dysthymia is known as "double depression." *DSM-IV*, 346.
2. René J. Muller, "Karen Horney's 'Resigned Person' Heralds DSM-III-R's BPD," *Comprehensive Psychiatry* 34 (1993): 264–272.
3. But this time the abandonment was by the father, not the mother, as is posited by Masterson in his psychodynamic formulation of the etiology of borderline personality disorder (James F. Masterson, *Psychotherapy of the Borderline Adult: A Developmental Approach* [New York: Brunner/Mazel, 1976]).
4. James F. Masterson, *The Narcissistic and Borderline Disorders* (New York: Brunner/Mazel, 1981), pp. 187–188.
5. René J. Muller, *Anatomy of a Splitting Borderline: Description and Analysis of a Case History* (Westport, CT: Praeger, 1994).
6. *DSM-IV*, 328–332; 335–338.
7. Caroline Kettlewell, *Skin Game* (New York: St. Martin's Press, 1999); and Steven Levenkron, *Cutting: Understanding and Overcoming Self-Mutilation* (New York: W.W. Norton, 1998).
8. Simon A. Grolnick, *The Work & Play of Winnicott* (Northvale, NJ: Jason Aronson, 1990), pp. 30–31.
9. Kay Redfield Jamison, *An Unquiet Mind: A Memoir of Moods and Madness* (New York: Alfred A. Knopf, 1995).
10. Ross J. Baldessarini, "A Plea for Integrity of the Bipolar Disorder Concept," *Bipolar Disorder* 2 (2000): 3–7.

11. Saying that someone has a personality disorder does not necessarily imply a compromised brain structure and function (Kenneth R. Silk, Ed., *Biology of Personality Disorders. Review of Psychiatry*, Vol. 17 [Washington, DC: American Psychiatric Association Press, 1998]; and Kenneth R. Silk, Ed., *Biological and Neurobehavioral Studies of Borderline Personality Disorder* [Washington, DC: American Psychiatric Association Press, 1994]).
12. René J. Muller, "To Understand Depression, Look to Psychobiology, not Biopsychiatry," *Psychiatric Times* (August 2003): 43–46.
13. K. Michael Lipkin, Jarl Dyrud, and George G Meyer, "The Many Faces of Mania: Therapeutic Trial of Lithium Carbonate," *Archives of General Psychiatry* 22 (1970): 262–267.
14. David S. Janowsky, Melitta Leff, and Richard S. Epstein, "Playing the Manic Game: Interpersonal Maneuvers of the Acutely Manic Patient," *Archives of General Psychiatry* 22 (1970): 252–261.
15. Baldessarini, "A Plea for Integrity"; see also Ross J. Baldessarini, "Fifty Years of Biomedical Psychiatry and Psychopharmcology in America," in Roy W. Menninger and John C. Nemiah, Eds., *Fifty Years of American Psychiatry, a Volume Celebrating the 150th Anniversary of the American Psychiatric Association* (Washington, DC: American Psychiatric Association Press, 1999).
16. Baldessarini, "A Plea for Integrity," p. 5.
17. Muller, *Beyond Marginality*, p. 50: "In Descartes's *Cogito*, the world becomes what I think about the world and how the world is reconstructed in my mind. The ego takes over for the self, becoming self-absorbed. Husserl, and the more existentially oriented phenomenologists who followed him, give the intellect back to the world, reestablishing the link Descartes cut. They use the word intentionality to name this connection of person to world, and to specify the direction of consciousness turned toward the world, rather than inward on itself."
18. Margaret Talbot, "The Bad Mother: Munchausen Syndrome by Proxy Is a Rare, Bizarre Disorder. Why Are So Many Women Being Accused of It?" *New Yorker*, August 9 & 16, 2004, 63–75.
19. "Manic-like episodes that are clearly caused by somatic antidepressant treatment (e.g., medication, electroconvulsive therapy, light therapy) should not count toward a diagnosis of Bipolar I Disorder" (*DSM-IV*, 332).
20. Cited in Joan Acocella, "Blocked: Why Do Writers Stop Writing?" *New Yorker*, June 14 & 21, 2004, 110–129. "Once you invent a category ... people will sort themselves into it, behave according to the description, and thus contrive new ways of being."

Chapter 7: Willing Psychotic Symptoms

The first section of this chapter, the story of Mrs. K, was published earlier (René J. Muller, "Willing Paranoid Delusions," *Psychiatric Times* [December 2006]: 33–35).

1. David J. Gerber and Susumu Tonegawa, "Psychotomimetic Effects of Drugs—A Common Pathway to Schizophrenia?" *New England Journal of Medicine* 350 (2004): 1047–1048.

2. Mrs. K's story reminds us that the community provides many chances for the attuned clinician to observe interesting and challenging psychopathology *in situ*.
3. *DSM-IV*, 296–301.
4. John Milton, *The Complete Poetry of John Milton*, Ed. John T. Shawcross (New York: Doubleday, 1971), Book I, Verse 1, Lines 254–255.
5. Heidegger, *Being and Time*.
6. Philippa A. Garety, "Making Sense of Delusions," *Psychiatry* 55 (1992): 282–291; see also Larry Davidson, "Commentary on Garety," 292–296.
7. John Perry, "Treating First-Break Psychosis in a Non-Hospital Environment," Department of Psychiatry Seminar, The Johns Hopkins University School of Medicine, March 26, 1990.
8. *The Collected Works of C.G. Jung: The Psychogenesis of Mental Disease*, Vol. 3, Eds. Herbert Read, Michael Fordham, Gerhard Adler, Trans. R.F.C. Hull (Princeton, NJ: Princeton University Press, 1960), p. 189.
9. R.D. Laing, *The Divided Self*.
10. R.D. Laing, *The Politics of Experience* (New York: Ballantine Books, 1967), p. 115.
11. Nigel J. Blackwood, Robert J. Howard, Richard P. Bentall, and Robin M. Murray, "Cognitive Neuropsychiatric Models of Persecutory Delusions," *American Journal of Psychiatry* 158 (2001): 527–539.
12. Sylvia Nasar, *A Beautiful Mind: The Life of Mathematical Genius and Nobel Laureate John Nash* (New York: Simon & Schuster, 1998).
13. Dana Kennedy, "The Mind Inside the Madness," *The New York Times*, April 21, 2002, Sec. 2.
14. J.H. van den Berg, *A Different Existence: Principles of Phenomenological Psychopathology* (Pittsburgh: Duquesne University Press, 1972).
15. In other words, from a highly abstract realm far removed from what most people would consider everyday reality. The chess master Bobby Fischer has spent his life in another kind of highly rarefied atmosphere, where the tendency toward abstraction is compounded by the kind of cutthroat competition that can incline one toward paranoia. See the brief, insightful essay on Bobby Fischer by Charles Krauthammer, "Did Chess Make Him Crazy?" *Time*, May 2, 2005, 96.
16. Nasar, p. 335.
17. Caryn James, "The Man, Not the Legend, of 'A Beautiful Mind'," *The New York Times*, April 26, 2002, B28.
18. Nasar, p. 358.
19. Ibid., p. 351.
20. *DSM-II*, 36. See also Jane Simpson and D. John Done, "Elasticity and Confabulation in Schizophrenic Delusions," *Psychological Medicine* 32 (2002): 451–458.
21. Andreasen, *Brave New Brain*, p. 183.
22. In addition to Laing see Breggin, *Toxic Psychiatry*. Breggin describes a condition he calls "schizophrenic" overwhelm, which can look like schizophrenia but is really extreme anxiety.
23. Richard P. Bentall, Gillian Haddock, and Peter D. Slade, "Cognitive Behavior Therapy for Persistent Auditory Hallucinations: From Theory to Therapy," *Behavior Therapy* 25 (1994): 51–66. In *Muses, Madmen, and Prophets: Rethinking the History, Science, and Meaning of Auditory*

Hallucination (New York: The Penguin Press, 2007), Daniel B. Smith shows how "voice-hearing" was considered a normal occurrence in past cultures and how what we now call auditory hallucinations can, in some instances, be explained psychodynamically.
24. Cited in Margo Jefferson, "I Wish I Had Said That, and I Will," *The New York Times Book Review*, April 11, 2004, 23.
25. Quoted in Claire Messud's review of Victoria Glendinning's *Leonard Woolf: A Biography* (New York: Free Press, 2006), *The New York Times Book Review*, December 10, 2006, 16.

Chapter 8: How Psychiatry Does Depression Wrong

1. In *Prozac Backlash*, Glenmullen describes what he calls the "mystique of a biochemical imbalance," pp. 195–198.
2. Matthew S. Milak, Ramin V. Parsey, John Keilp, Maria A. Oquendo, Kevin M. Malone, and J. John Mann, "Neuroanatomic Correlates of Psychopathologic Components of Major Depressive Disorder," *Archives of General Psychiatry* 62 (2005): 397–408; John Medina, "What PET Scans Actually Measure," *Psychiatric Times* (November 1999): 93–95; and Nora D. Volkow and Laurence R. Tancredi, "Biological Correlates of Mental Activity Studied with PET," *American Journal of Psychiatry* 148 (1991): 439–443.
3. Paul R. McHugh and Phillip R. Slavney, *The Perspectives of Psychiatry, Second Edition*, (Baltimore: The Johns Hopkins University Press, 1998).
4. Ibid., p. 12.
5. Jonathan Franzen, *The Corrections* (New York: Farrar, Straus and Giroux, 2001), p. 318.
6. Ibid., p. 319.
7. Ibid., p. 322.
8. Kramer, *Listening to Prozac*, pp. 1–21.
9. Glenmullen vividly describes many different kinds of adverse reactions he has seen in his own patients, as well as those reported in journal articles by other clinicians.
10. Glenmullen, *Prozac Backlash*, p. 214.
11. Ibid., pp. 64–78.
12. Michael Babyak, James A. Blumenthal, Steve Herman, Parinda Khatri, Murali Doraiswamy, Kathleen Moore, Edward Craighead, Teri T. Baldewicz, and K. Ranga Krishnan, "Exercise Treatment for Major Depression: Maintenance of Therapeutic Benefit at 10 Months," *Psychosomatic Medicine* 62 (2000): 633–638.
13. David O. Antonuccio, William G. Danton, and G.Y. DeNelsky, "Psychotherapy Versus Medication for Depression: Challenging the Conventional Wisdom With Data," *Professional Psychology: Research and Practice* 26 (1995): 574–585.
14. Irving Kirsch and David Antonuccio, "Antidepressants Versus Placebos: Meaningful Advantages are Lacking," *Psychiatric Times* (September 2002): 6–8. Counterpoint response: Michael E. Thase, "Small Effects Are Not Trivial from a Public Health Perspective," *Psychiatric Times* (September

2002): 9. See also: P. Hazell, D. O'Connell, D. Heathcote, J. Robertson, and D. Henry, "Efficacy of Tricyclic Drugs in Treating Child and Adolescent Depression: A Meta-Analysis," *British Medical Journal* 310 (1995): 897–901.

In 1995, psychiatrist Colin A. Ross and psychologist Alvin Pam published *Pseudoscience in Biological Psychiatry: Blaming the Body* (New York: John Wiley & Sons, 1995), which pulled no punches in showing how data from the journal articles that are most frequently cited in formulating the "science" of biological psychiatry were derived, empirically and statistically. Ross and Pam insist that most of the inferences drawn from these data were the result of poor thinking and bad statistical analysis. See Jonathan P. Schindelheim's review, *New England Journal of Medicine* 332 (1995): 1795–1796.

15. In *Psych ER: Psychiatric Patients Come to the Emergency Room*, I explored, using Jean-Paul Sartre's ontology, that idea that, in the face of a negative experience, a person can, rather than overcome the loss, give in to it and de-differentiate his world to the point where what the world continues to offer is deliberately refused. I argue that this refusal *itself* constitutes the meaning and structure of what we call depression (*Psych ER*, pp. 3–10). See also René J. Muller, "To Understand Depression, Look to Psychobiology, Not Biopsychiatry," *Psychiatric Times* (August 2003): 41–46; René J. Muller, "Brain Changes and Placebo" (letter), *American Journal of Psychiatry* 160 (2003): 389–390; and "Comment," 390–391.

Chapter 9: Saving Psychiatry From the Brain

1. Benjamin Carson, "Your Mind Can Map Your Destiny," *Parade*, December 7, 2003, 28–30.
2. Jean-Paul Sartre, *Nausea*, p. 99.
3. George E. Vaillant, "The Beginning of Wisdom Is Never Calling a Patient a Borderline," Department of Psychiatry Seminar, University of Maryland School of Medicine, March 3, 1990. At that time, Professor Vaillant also went on record as believing, "We call borderlines borderlines because we do not have the courage to call them assholes."
4. David L. Rosenhan, "On Being Sane in Insane Places," *Science* 179 (1973): 250–258.
5. Andreasen, *Brave New Brain*, p. 3.
6. Peter J. Manos, "The Utility of the Ten-Point Clock Test as a Screen for Cognitive Impairment in General Hospital Patients," *General Hospital Psychiatry* 19 (1997): 439–444.
7. Paul R. McHugh, "Psychiatric Misadventures," *The American Scholar* 61 (1992): 497–510.

Chapter 10: Doing Psychiatry Right

1. Rosenhan, "On Being Sane in Insane Places," 257.
2. Quoted in Benedict Carey, "Can Brain Scans See Depression?" *The New York Times*, October 18, 2005, D1, D6.

3. John Horgan, *The End of Science: Facing the Limits of Knowledge in the Twilight of the Scientific Age* (New York: Broadway Books, 1996). See also John Horgan, "In Defense of Common Sense," *The New York Times*, August 12, 2005, A19: "I have also found common sense—ordinary, nonspecialized knowledge and judgment—to be indispensable for judging scientists' pronouncements, even, or especially, in the most esoteric fields." Simply put, much of what is offered now as "proof" for the hegemony of the brain in determining human thought, emotion, and behavior defies the intuitive, common-sense approach to life accumulated over centuries. The quintessential natural scientist Albert Einstein noted, "The intuitive mind is a sacred gift and the rational mind is a faithful servant. We have created a society that honors the servant and has forgotten the gift." Quoted in Ronald Pies, "The Rabbi's Brain: Did a 19th Century Mystic Anticipate Modern Neurobiology?" *Psychiatric Times* (September 2005): 63–64.
4. John Eccles, *How the Self Controls Its Brain* (Berlin: Springer-Verlag, 1994). "In formulating more precisely the dualist hypothesis of mind-brain interaction, the initial statement is that the whole world of mental events has an existence as autonomous as the world of matter-energy," p. 106.
5. This was the intuition experienced by the 10-year-old Benjamin Carson, who went on to become a renowned neurosurgeon, as he looked at a drawing of a human brain and realized that, unlike the brains of animals, we have frontal lobes that allow us to directly participate in our own fate. See the beginning of Chapter 9.
6. Jeffrey Kluger (with reporting by Jeff Chu, Broward Liston, Maggie Sieger, and Daniel Williams), "Is God in Our Genes?" *Time*, October 25, 2004, 62–72.
7. Dean Hamer, *The God Gene: How Faith Is Hard-Wired Into Our Genes* (New York: Doubleday, 2004).
8. John Tierney, "Using MRIs to See Politics on the Brain," *The New York Times*, Tuesday, April 20, 2004, A1, A17.
9. Jim Holt, "Of Two Minds: Are We Sure We Really Want to Know How the Brain Functions?" *The New York Times Magazine*, May 8, 2005, 11–13. The journal article Holt commented on is Yukiyasu Kamitani and Frank Tong, "Decoding the Visual and Subjective Contents of the Human Brain," *Nature Neuroscience* 8 (2005): 679–685.
10. Jean-Paul Sartre, *Existentialism and Human Emotions*, Trans. Bernard Frechtman and Hazel E. Barnes (New York: Philosophical Library, 1957).
11. Harper, *The Existential Experience*; see also Ralph Harper, *On Presence: Variations and Reflections* (Baltimore: The Johns Hopkins University Press, 2006).
12. Ludwig Binswanger, *Being-in-the-World: Selected Papers of Ludwig Binswanger*, Trans. Jacob Needleman (New York: Harper & Row, 1963); Medard Boss, *Psychoanalysis and Daseinanalysis*, Trans. Ludwig B. Lefebre (New York: Basic Books, 1963); Karl Jaspers: *General Psychopathology*, Vol. 1, Trans. J. Hoenig and Marian W. Hamilton, with a new foreword by Paul R. McHugh (Baltimore: The Johns Hopkins University Press, 1997); Viktor E. Frankl: *Man's Search for Meaning: An Introduction to Logotherapy*, part one, Trans.

Ilse Lasch, with a preface by Gordon W. Allport (New York: Pocket Books, 1963); J.H. van den Berg: *A Different Existence: Principles of Phenomenological Psychopathology* (Pittsburgh: Duquesne University Press, 1972).

13. Philippe Pinel (1806), *A Treatise on Insanity*, Section 1, Trans. D.D. David (New York: Hafner Publishing, 1962, for the Library of the New York Academy of Medicine; cited in *Psychiatric Times*, Bipolar Disorder & Impulse Spectrum Letter [August, 2001]: 8).
14. Robert Stone, "The Villains," *The New York Times Magazine*, September 23, 2001, 22.
15. Aaron T. Beck, *Cognitive Therapy and the Emotional Disorders* (New York: International Universities Press, 1976); and Jerome D. Frank and Julia B. Frank, *Persuasion and Healing: A Comparative Study of Psychotherapy*, 3rd ed. (Baltimore: The Johns Hopkins University Press, 1991).
16. Muller, *Psych ER*, pp. 159–166.
17. Karl Jaspers, *Philosophy*, Vol. 2 (Chicago: University of Chicago Press, 1977), pp. 177–223.
18. Otto F. Kernberg, Michael A. Selzer, Harold W. Koenigsberg, Arthur C. Carr, and Ann H. Appelbaum, *Psychodynamic Psychotherapy of Borderline Patients* (New York: Basic Books, 1989); see also Muller, *Anatomy of a Splitting Borderline.*
19. This and the next quote in the same paragraph are from Paul R. McHugh, "Beyond the *DSM-IV*: From Appearances to Essences," *Psychiatric Research Report*, Vol. 17 (Summer 2001): 2–3 and 14–15. The text may be found at http://hopkinsmedicine.org/press/2001/august/McHugh.htm
20. Ibid., p. 4.
21. Theodore Lidz, "Adolf Meyer and the Development of American Psychiatry," *American Journal of Psychiatry* 123 (1966), 320–332.
22. Genova, "Dump the DSM!" For a beautifully written account of the current state of psychiatry see Paul Genova, *The Thaw: Reclaiming the Person for Psychiatry*, 2nd ed. (Hillsdale, NJ: The Analytic Press, 2002).
23. Ralph D. Ellis, "Phenomenology-Friendly Neuroscience: The Return to Merleau-Ponty as Psychologist," *Human Studies* 29 (2006), 33–55; and Maurice Merleau-Ponty, *The Structure of Behavior*, Trans. Alden L. Fisher (Boston: Beacon Press, 1967).
24. The "top-down/bottom-up" terminology is derived from the biopsychosocial model of mental illness proposed by George L. Engel (George L. Engel, "The Clinical Application of the Biopsychosocial Model," *American Journal of Psychiatry* 137 [1980]: 535–544); see also Alfred M. Freedman, "The Biopsychosocial Paradigm and the Future of Psychiatry," *Comprehensive Psychiatry* 36 (1995): 397–404; and Larry Davidson and John S. Strauss, "Beyond the Biopsychosocial Model: Integrating Disorder, Health, and Recovery," *Psychiatry* 58 (1995): 44–55.

    I have made my own attempt at a "top-down/bottom-up," psychobiological synthesis, proposing an association between the brain lateralization of negative experience and a primitive defense known as *splitting*. See René J. Muller, "Is There a Neural Basis for Borderline Splitting?" *Comprehensive Psychiatry* 33 (1992): 92–104. The placebo effect is the ultimate mind-brain, psychobiological response. This phenomenon, which is increasingly being recognized for its strength and generality, demonstrates the active, ongoing capacity of consciousness, in conjunction with a complementary neural substrate, to construct human experience. See René J. Muller, "Brain Changes and Placebo," *American Journal of Psychiatry* 160 (2003): 389–390 (letter).

Index

M

T

U

V

W

X

Y

Z